_Advantage_

"The need for nurses to be savvy online is just as important as being literate. _The Nurse's Social Media Advantage_ will propel a new breed of nurses who can intelligently share their experiences, collaborate with other health care professionals, and more easily make the difference in patients' lives that all nurses hope to do."

–Phil Baumann, BSN, RN
Founder, HealthIsSocial.com, RNchat, and MDchat
Advisory Board Member, Mayo Clinic Center for Social Media

"If the words social media sound like words from another language, then this book will serve as a translation tool. It contains clear, concise explanations and direction to navigate your way into the exciting and absorbing world of social media and social networking."

–Judith Shamian PhD, RN, FAAN
President and CEO, VON Canada
President, Canadian Nurses Association

"Here comes the future, so get with it! Rob Fraser's *The Nurse's Social Media Advantage* will be your guide to the universe of social media in your nursing practice."

–Mary Ferguson-Paré, PhD, RN, CHE
Vice President, Professional Affairs and Chief Nurse Executive
University Health Network
Toronto

"*The Nurse's Social Media Advantage* is a must-have book for nurses who want to get up to speed with current technology. Rob Fraser walks us through the basics of how to be tech-savvy health care professionals, whether from a home laptop, a work computer on a nursing unit, or a smart phone. Throughout the book, he emphasizes patient confidentiality, privacy, and advocacy, as well as how to promote the nursing profession through the contribution of our own best practices and knowledge."

–Patrick Hickey, DrPH, RN, CNOR
Clinical Assistant Professor
University of South Carolina College of Nursing
Author, *7 Summits: A Nurse's Quest to Conquer Mountaineering and Life*

The Nurse's Social Media Advantage

How Making Connections and Sharing Ideas Can Enhance Your Nursing Career

By Robert Fraser, BScN, RN
@rdjfraser

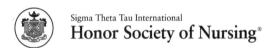

Sigma Theta Tau International
Honor Society of Nursing

Sigma Theta Tau International

The Honor Society of Nursing, Sigma Theta Tau International, the only international honor society worldwide, is a global community of nurse leaders with members who live in 86 countries and belong to 469 chapters. Through this network, members lead in using knowledge, scholarship, service, and learning to improve the health of the world's people.

Sigma Theta Tau International
550 West North Street
Indianapolis, IN 46202

To order additional books, buy in bulk, or order for corporate use, contact Nursing Knowledge International at 888.NKI.4YOU (888.654.4968/US and Canada) or +1.317.634.8171 (outside US and Canada).

To request a review copy for course adoption, e-mail solutions@nursingknowledge.org or call 888.NKI.4YOU (888.654.4968/US and Canada) or +1.317.917.4983 (outside US and Canada).

To request author information, or for speaker or other media requests, contact Rachael McLaughlin of the Honor Society of Nursing, Sigma Theta Tau International at 888.634.7575 (US and Canada) or +1.317.634.8171 (outside US and Canada).

Print ISBN-13:   978-1-935476-01-6
EPUB ISBN: 978-1-935476-34-4
PDF ISBN: 978-1-935476-35-1

Library of Congress Cataloging-in-Publication Data

Fraser, Robert, 1986-
   The nurse's social media advantage : how making connections and sharing ideas can enhance your nursing practice / Robert Fraser.
       p. ; cm.
   Includes bibliographical references.
   ISBN 978-1-935476-01-6 (alk. paper)
   1. Nursing informatics. 2. Medical care--Computer network resources. 3. Internet. I. Sigma Theta Tau International. II. Title.
   [DNLM: 1. Internet. 2. Nursing. 3. Communications Media. 4. Information Dissemination--methods. WY 26.5]
   RT50.5.F73 2011
   610.730285--dc22

                                        2011004537

First Printing, 2011

Publisher: Renee Wilmeth
Principal Editor: Carla Hall
Development Editor/Copy Editor: Kate Shoup
Proofreader: Jane Palmer
Interior Design and Page Composition: Rebecca Batchelor

Acquisitions Editor: Janet Boivin, RN
Project Editor: Billy Fields
Editorial Coordinator: Paula Jeffers
Cover Designer: Studio Galou
Indexer: Johnna Van Hoose Dinse

Dedication

This book is dedicated to Dianne Martin and Laurie Clune. Dianne is the reason I love my career and the person who influenced my decision to become a nurse. I cannot thank her enough for her constant guidance and support in nursing. Laurie was the professor who pushed me to write my first conference abstract, which caused me to fall down the rabbit hole of social media in nursing. I enjoyed her class, but it was this life lesson for which I will be forever in her debt. Thanks to both of them for their love of our profession, their leadership in nursing, and the impact they have made on me and countless others.

Acknowledgements

There is no way I could have done anything that I have accomplished without my parents, Jim and Donna Fraser. For your love and support, I truly thank you. David Ramjattan was the first person to listen to my questions and give me thoughtful answers. Our conversations took my mind to places I had never been, long before he helped me travel the world.

Linda Cooper was the first professor to inspire me upon entering nursing school, and certainly not the last. I have always been blessed with phenomenal career and leadership advice from so many people, including Janice Waddell, Margareth Zanchetta, and Nancy Walton. I thank you all for your feedback, support, and continual encouragement.

This book would not have been possible without a number of people. Thanks to each and every one who contributed. I could have never guessed where Elliot Pesut's e-mail to connect me with Sigma Theta Tau International (STTI) and Dan Pesut would take me, or that Jane Palmer's kind phone calls and hospitality would help me work so closely with STTI. From my first introduction, I have been continually astonished at the friendly and enthusiastic staff who helped me to get this book onto the page. Thank you Janet Boivin, Carla Hall, Renee Wilmeth, Kate Shoup, Jane Palmer, and Billy Fields for your constant support and constructive comments throughout the process!

Finally, I have to thank Joanna Fraser and Alanna Fennell: Your small acts of kindness and large acts of encouragement helped me make it through, from the first sentence to the last.

About the Author

Robert Fraser, BScN, RN | Learn more, help others.
http://nursingideas.ca | http://nurserob.com
contact@robertfraser.ca | @rdjfraser

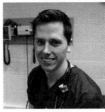 Robert Fraser, BScN, RN, is a nurse who is passionate about how technology can change the way we share information. He is an active and engaged individual, both at home and abroad. Locally, he has volunteered in a number of places, from soup kitchens to health care advisory boards. Regionally, Fraser has advised the Registered Nurses' Association of Ontario on digital strategy. Nationally, he has been involved in student groups and worked with nursing-advocacy groups. Internationally, he has worked on community-development projects in Trinidad and Tobago, Germany, and India.

Fraser's creativity and interest in technology became an important part of his nursing career when he was an undergraduate. In 2008, he launched Nursing Ideas (http://nursingideas.ca), an online nursing repository for connecting nurses and nursing students with leaders, innovators, and researchers in health care. Video interviews with guests have ranged from Marla Salmon, former chief nurse of the United States, to journalist and nursing advocate Suzanne Gordon. The website has attracted more than 25,000 visitors from 118 countries, which has validated Fraser's belief that nurses can benefit from using technology and online tools.

After finishing his undergraduate degree at Ryerson University, Fraser was recruited to complete his Master of Nursing degree at the University of Toronto and expects to graduate in the summer of 2011. He was the only nurse to be selected for an Innovation (isuma) Fellowship to work with the Health Strategy Innovation Cell, an advisory research group for the Ontario Ministry of Health. Currently, he is a Junior Fellow at Massey College and working with health care organizations to better engage patients and providers online.

Table of Contents

Foreword

Rob Fraser is passionate about nursing and social media. No wonder he managed to write a book in which his passion for social media makes a significant contribution in supporting the knowledge, skills, and abilities of professional nursing colleagues around the world.

My own acquaintance with Rob is a product of social networking. A few years ago, I was consulting at Arizona State University, where I met nurse colleague Daniel Weberg. It just so happens that my son, Elliott, was with me at the time. Elliott was doing online courseware for an airline. I invited him to participate in the consultation project, because of his experiences with simulation in the aviation industry. Elliott ended up linking with Daniel through Twitter. Daniel then linked Elliott with Rob Fraser—who, at that time, was a nursing student in Canada. Before long, Elliott linked Rob to me. So, a nursing colleague in Arizona became part of my son's social network, resulting in a nursing student in Canada being linked to my son—who, in turn, linked the nursing student with a past president of the Honor Society of Nursing, Sigma Theta Tau International (STTI), the publisher of this book. This example illustrates the power and potential of social media and the influence and effect of social networking.

Over time, I engaged in several e-mail conversations with Rob. I learned more about him and admired and appreciated his work documenting his interviews with nursing leaders. I encouraged him to submit an abstract for STTI's 2009 Biennial Convention, and his abstract on social media was accepted. I also linked him with several honor society staff—I know exceptional talent when I see it! Rob traveled to Indiana, where we had a great face-to-face meeting. He presented his work to a room packed full of colleagues. He even videotaped his presentation; it's posted at http://www.viddler.com/explore/rfraser/videos/49/. He also took time at that convention to interview several other nursing leaders and capture their wisdom on video. Since that time, Rob has continued to use his knowledge, skills, and intelligence—as well as his wit and charm—to advance his interests in nursing, innovation, leadership influence, and the power of social media to make a difference for nurses and patients and to create a better world. And now, he has authored a book on the subject.

(Editor's note: Rob's social network ultimately brought him to the attention of STTI editors. While this theory may not be scientifically provable, we believe that without Rob's social media connections, we would not have found him to write this book.)

If you are new to social media or want to know more about it, this book is an excellent introduction. Here you are likely to discover how best to classify yourself in the world of social media. Are you an Inactive? Spectator? Joiner? Collector? Critic? Creator? Rob uses the nursing process to explain and evaluate the do's and don'ts of social media for nurses. In a simple, direct, and straightforward way, he explains the functions, purpose, capabilities, and potentials associated with evaluating websites. He clearly explains industry standards for social media and provides examples of his favorite tools and resources.

Read this book and you will understand the power and promise of social media for building your professional reputation and profile. You will learn to create and sustain social networks to advance your personal and professional interests. You are likely to discover new ways of staying informed and connecting with colleagues who share your passions. You will discover new ways of linking and communicating with others through online communities of practice. Most importantly, Rob discusses how best to manage the risks and liabilities of social media through smart decision making.

He provides guidance and tips to help you navigate the complexities of social media. In fact, he makes complex ideas simple. For example, in exploring the world of social media, he advises each of us to be transparent, accurate, considerate, generous, and a good participant. He also tells nurses to uphold professional, organizational, and personal values; respect copyright laws; and keep confidential information confidential!

He also challenges each of us to maintain our curiosity and learn. Life-long learning is a core professional nursing responsibility and value. Learning about emerging technologies is challenging for all of us. However, as he observes, it is not really about the technology: Rather, it is about how you can use the technology to enhance your knowledge, skills, abilities, and understandings to connect with people and build relationships that create community—and inspire people to make a difference in the world through personal and professional action.

After reading this book, you will have new appreciation for the tools and services that are available to you through the Internet. As Rob notes, the Internet is yet another way that nurses can build relationships, create content, find and share information, collaborate with others, and create a global nursing knowledge network.

Enjoy your exploration and learning. And thank you, Rob Fraser, for being the next-generation nursing leader that you are.

—Daniel J. Pesut, PhD, RN, PMHCNS-BC, FAAN
Past President (2003-05)
Honor Society of Nursing, Sigma Theta Tau International
Professor of Nursing
Indiana University School of Nursing
Indianapolis, Indiana, USA

Introduction

Most people assume when they hear about the latest gadget, invention, or late-breaking piece of news that it is brand new, something completely different. This is especially true with social media. In fact, social media is simply an evolution in communication technology.

Even experts have different thoughts on the exact definition of social media. The most concise and easy to grasp—as well as my favorite—is a 2008 Wikipedia definition that described social media as "primarily Internet- and mobile-based tools for sharing and discussing information among human beings." Looking at this definition, it's easy to see that social media is all about sharing and discussing information.

Before social media, humans used hieroglyphs, tablets, parchment, books, and eventually radio and video to communicate. Anyone who consumed these sources of information could then share what they learned through discussion (face-to-face, letters, over the phone, etc.), by giving other people the media (surrendering their copy, photocopying, e-mailing, making a mix tape, etc.) or by creating their own media to include their own thoughts (research papers, books, magazine articles, etc.). Now we have a whole host of new ways to create, store, and share information, as well as new ways to participate, interact, and discuss this media. These aren't time-wasting activities; they are a whole new set of tools!

Another way to grasp the term social media is by breaking it apart. The phrase really combines social networking and new media. In the past, social networks were built slowly by meeting new people and exchanging phone numbers, e-mail addresses, and maybe even business cards. As technology has evolved, however, so have the ways in which we can meet people, exchange information, and maintain relationships. Now, we don't have to carry around an address book in our pockets; our directory is updated whenever someone updates his or her profile on LinkedIn. Now, e-mail has provided a new option; we can send a message without buying stamps, waiting for a mail carrier, and worrying whether our friend will get it. This doesn't mean we never see our friends in person; these new options just make it easier to keep up to date with their changing lives and get in touch with them when we need to.

The way we manage relationships is not the only thing that has changed. Media has also seen dramatic changes. There is no way our parents could have afforded to make, edit, and distribute a high definition video when they were kids. It didn't even exist when they were kids. As technology becomes cheaper and easier to use, more people can participate. A plethora of new media is being posted on sites such as YouTube (http://youtube.com) and created by web services such as Animoto (http://animoto.com)—free, no less. Traditional types of media limited individuals' ability to choose, because they were the only choice. New media empowers individuals to create content related to their expertise, contribute to their own social groups, and find information tailored to their interests.

Maybe you feel like this is too much—you already have too many relationships to manage and you're already overloaded with information, so why do you need social media too? There are two reasons. To start, it is not going anywhere. Social media—the way we communicate and share ideas—will continue to evolve, whether nurses get involved or not. The only risk is that our profession will be left behind. More importantly, social media is about new tools and services. This is the reason I get excited, and other nurses should too. Social media provides new possibilities for building relationships, creating content, finding and sharing information, and collaborating with others.

Social media is here to stay, and nurses need to understand how to use it. The intent of this book is to explain how the Internet has changed and how nurses need to shift their thinking and use of digital toolsets accordingly. By the end of this book, you should be able to do the following:

* Explain social media to others.

* Build your professional profile, reputation, and network online.

* Find others who share your interests.

* Participate in online communities.

* Manage the risks and liability of social media by making smart decisions.

Key Features

Each chapter begins by asking the reader *Do you know ...* questions.

Following the tradition of the *Nurse's Advantage* books, a "question and answer" format is used to enable you to target what you need or want to learn.

Insights and Inspirations

Talking about social media without mentioning how others have used it makes as much sense as selling a car without an engine. "Insights and Inspirations" is a section to introduce you to nurses who have been inspired by social media and to provide you with a short lesson or bit of advice.

TIP
Tips highlight important points to remember.

Tables and figures have been included to help illustrate and better explain key topics.

⑤ This is what a table will look like in the book	
Column 1 Heading	**Column 2 Heading**
Column 1 data will be here	Column 2 data will be here

Whether talking on the unit, by the water cooler, or at conferences, nurses have a lot of questions about social media.

A frequently asked questions section appears at the end of some chapters to help answer those questions directly.

I love books, but they do not do justice to the Internet. To bring the chapters to life, there are exercises to complete at the end. Don't worry; they don't involve calculus. The exercises are just some simple instructions to help you think about and observe what was talked about in the chapter.

Quiz

1. True or false: Nurses are not allowed to participate in social media online due to confidentiality.

> **False:** Nurses are allowed to participate in online communities. However, they must adhere to the same professional codes of conduct that govern any communications, which means adhering to confidentiality guidelines.

2. True or false: My hospital blocks social-networking sites. Therefore, there is no point in my using them.

> **False**. If your hospital has blocked social-networking sites, investigate whether they have other policies for employees using social media. These rules are important to follow, but they do not mean you cannot create a professional profile for networking or share information for which you take responsibility.

3. True or false: Social media will take a lot of my time.

> **False**. What takes time is learning how these tools work. When you can make an informed decision about how you want to use these tools, there is a great deal of variability on how much time you need to invest.

4. True or false: Nurses are increasingly using social media sites, so I can benefit from participating too.

> **True.** Nurses are slowly adopting more online tools as they find out their uses. That means there are likely services that you could benefit from using. Also, participating in dialogue with other professionals interested in a particular topic is a great way to network.

A. Collaborate on documents

B. Make slideshows

C. Post your résumé

D. Watch videos

C: Post your résumé. LinkedIn is a professional networking site that enables you to list your education, work, and professional experiences. It also lets you add connections and manage your contacts.

A. Host a website

B. Post PowerPoint presentations

C. Find pictures

D. Share large files

B: Post PowerPoint presentations. SlideShare lets users share slides and record audio files to go with presentations. Nurses can share information for patients, other providers, or students in this way.

True. Short URLs were created to enable users to share URLs within Twitter messages, which must be less than 140 characters. However, they are usually much shorter. Short URLs are also useful because they enable users to create easy-to-remember URLs and track how many people access them.

A. Find amusing videos

B. Post educational material

C. Promote yourself

D. All of the above

D: All of the above. There are many uses for YouTube, such as finding a video to illustrate a point in a presentation. YouTube can also be a great way to share and find information, and to market your expertise.

9. True or false: Once you have learned the most important social media tools, you will not have to learn anything else.

False. As you know from your nursing education, learning is never done. The same goes for social media. As your knowledge expands, the time required to learn a new tool should decrease. You will also develop a better ability to evaluate the potential usefulness of a tool for your purposes.

10. True or false: Nurses can lose their job or license for using social media inappropriately.

True. Although it is not fun to talk about, there are consequences for inappropriate use of social media. However, a little common sense and critical thinking go a long way! Nurses need to remember the professional standards they are accountable for, and that very little (if anything) of what is posted on the Internet is 100% private.

1

✳

Laying the Foundation

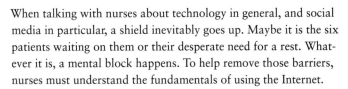

Do you:

Know how the Internet has changed?

Doubt that patients are using the Internet?

Understand how you can find specific types of content online?

Recognize the common icons that are appearing on different websites?

Feel you are a participant of the Internet?

When talking with nurses about technology in general, and social media in particular, a shield inevitably goes up. Maybe it is the six patients waiting on them or their desperate need for a rest. Whatever it is, a mental block happens. To help remove those barriers, nurses must understand the fundamentals of using the Internet.

From local and national news that affects nurses to the latest research and innovations in health care, nurses must, at a minimum, be able to access online resources, evaluate their validity, and integrate what they learn into their professional lives. But just as students learning math start with addition and subtraction before studying times tables, nurses must start with the basics when learning about the Internet and social media.

"It all depends on how we look at things, and not on how they are themselves."

–Carl Jung

Getting in the Right Mind-set

What are some reasons nurses don't want to learn social media?

Here are a few reasons nurses cite for avoiding social media:

* It is too difficult to learn.

* It takes too much time to learn and use.

* It won't help them.

* Its use is banned at their organization.

* Using social media means breaking patient confidentiality.

Is social media difficult to learn?

Social media is complex. But that's okay! There are few things worth knowing that are not complex. Remember your first biology textbook, with the illustrations and diagrams of blood vessels and lobes of lungs in the human anatomy? That information was complex, but you learned it. Similarly, social media can be learned; it just needs to be taught well. Besides, nursing work requires learning hundreds—if not thousands—of complex tasks. Compared to that, learning to use social media is nothing!

Does social media take too much time to learn and use?

No one can deny that learning takes time. However, time spent learning is time invested—and it will pay dividends in the long run. If you went to the library, you would not check every book's index or table of contents to determine whether it covered the topic you were researching. Rather, you would need to learn how to use the cataloging system to search for the appropriate resources, and how to effectively use those resources to save time. The same applies for social media: A better understanding of how to access knowledge online will save you time. Understanding the tools helps you selectively use your time and dedicate the minimum effort for maximum results.

Can social media help nurses?

Twitter may not be for everyone, but professional networking, sharing ideas, and collaboration are realities of the world you live in. Every nurse is different, and so will be the way he or she utilizes technology. That's OK. Once you learn about the various social media tools that are available, you can decide for yourself how to engage with those tools.

What if social media use is banned by your organization?

Facebook is now blocked in many hospital and community care centers, and Twitter may also be disallowed. That doesn't mean you can't use these tools; it simply means you need a different approach. Learn what the hospital's policies and expectations are, and then you can find ways to benefit from using social media tools while respecting your employer's rules. This may mean using social media outside of work hours.

Does using social media mean breaking patient confidentiality?

Social media changes what is public and private. For most of us, going to the grocery store is not on the record. But when Brad Pitt goes to the store, he might very well be videotaped or photographed.

For that reason, Pitt has had to learn to be careful what he says and does when he's in public. Similarly, nurses must learn what they can share, and where. Nurses are taught not to break patient confidentiality—but that doesn't mean nurses can't talk about work at home. Nurses who understand what information is being shared publicly and know how to appropriately talk about clinical experiences can contribute online and protect confidentiality at the same time.

How do you address doubts about learning social media?

Whether learning about the Internet, Twitter, or Facebook, you can easily let objections, doubts, and fears enter your mind. Instead, try to remember these things:

* Technology is not meant to be the focus. The idea is to connect with real people and make a real-world impact, such as improving practice or increasing knowledge sharing, that can help our careers and our patients.

* Time spent learning is time well-invested. Although media may change over time, what you learn will be helpful as technology and communication continue to evolve.

* Learning these tools can help you sort through information overload and share your knowledge, contribute to your career, and improve patients' lives.

* Social media is not about connecting to more people; it's about connecting with the right people—those who can benefit from your knowledge or share your interests.

* As a nurse, you learn to assess patients and identify opportunities to intervene, take action, and save lives. Learning a bit more about technology could not hurt, and sharing what you know will help both patients and the profession.

Learning about social media is like managing a savings account. Being consistent will bring results over time. Little by little, you will develop a wealth of knowledge. Once you have the right mind-set, you are ready for the basic building blocks.

"A mind, stretched to a new idea, never goes back to its original dimension."

—Oliver Wendell Holmes

Understanding the Internet

Do a lot of people use the Internet?

In a word, yes. According to the Pew Internet and American Life Project, 75% of adults and 95% of teenagers in the United States go online (Fox, 2008).

Why do nurses need to understand the Internet?

To understand how social media works, you need to understand what powers it: the Internet.

How did the Internet start?

The Internet isn't new. In fact, the Internet as we know it today has its roots in a computer network, ARPANET, that was created in 1969 to connect colleges, industry, and the U.S. Department of Defense. Over time, the Internet grew to include more and more computers. By 1987, there were roughly 10,000 computers connected to the Internet.

What is the World Wide Web?

Incompatibilities among protocols used to share data made navigating the burgeoning Internet problematic. In 1991, the development of the World Wide Web solved this problem. With the World Wide Web, anyone with a computer and a connection could access the Internet and view information (that is, content) in the form of a special document called a web page, using a special type of software called a web browser (Governor, Nickull, & Hinchcliffe, 2009; see

Figure 1.1). This original incarnation of the World Wide Web is often referred to as Web 1.0.

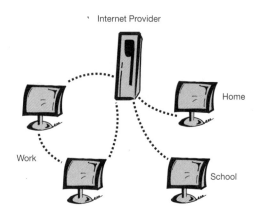

Figure 1.1: A simple illustration of a network.

How does the World Wide Web work?

In the early days of the Internet, documents were text only. Over time, however, standards for including pictures, audio, and video were developed. In addition, hyperlinks, now called links, were created to enable users to move from a web page on one web server (a computer where a web page is stored) to another page on that same server or on another server—even one on the other side of the globe! This enabled people to follow links that interested them and find other relevant web pages or websites. As the World Wide Web expanded, all types of media—print, radio, television— were added. People on the World Wide Web began to organize all sorts of information to serve a growing audience.

TIP As technology and tools became more accessible, wider participation became possible.

Why has the World Wide Web been successful?

The World Wide Web has been successful for a number of reasons:

* Anyone with a computer and a connection can participate.

* Users can call on information (in the form of web pages) whenever they want.

* Each web page has a unique web address (also called a URL, short for uniform resource locator) and can be linked to from other pages.

* Users can access information they are interested in—some of which they did not have access to before (resources were un-published, books and videos were too expensive or otherwise unavailable, etc.).

* Information can be delivered in a variety of formats.

* It allows for a personal experience. Individuals who know how to create their own pages can do so, and they can visit the pages of others.

> *"Advances in computer technology and the Internet have changed the way America works, learns, and communicates."*
>
> –Bill Clinton

What is Web 2.0?

Until the advent of the Internet and the World Wide Web, the way humans shared information had not seen a radical change since the debut of the Gutenberg printing press. That change didn't happen overnight, however. In the Web 1.0 phase, entities with websites were limited primarily to government organizations, colleges, uni-versities, and eventually mainstream organizations. Then, medium-sized and small businesses developed an online presence, along with a few individuals. In general, information traveled in one direction:

from the producer (the entity that supplied the web page) to the user (the person accessing the page), as shown in Figure 1.2. It wasn't until organizations began cultivating users, or consumers, as producers that the Web truly took off: eBay let users become sellers, MySpace let artists post music, Wikipedia let anyone edit an article, and Facebook let users share their thoughts with their online friends. (See Figure 1.3.). This shift is often referred to as Web 2.0.

"Web 2.0 and social media are today's printing press—changing society's relationships with computers and institutions, accelerating the spread of ideas, and influencing a collective determination of what's relevant and what's not."

–Francesca Barrientos and Elizabeth Foughty

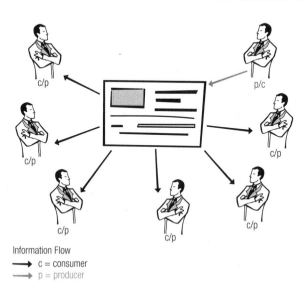

Information Flow
→ c = consumer
→ p = producer

Figure 1.2: Web 1.0—Producers and consumers.

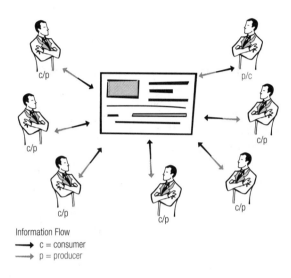

Figure 1.3: Web 2.0—Consumers become producers. (Inspired by Clay Shirky, 2009.)

If everyone can contribute, does that ruin the content?

Some users felt that having everyone jump the Internet bandwagon was akin to people crashing the party. Experts such as Tim O'Reilly (2005) disagreed, pointing out that this enables users to create, contribute, and form communities online.

Naturally, people tend to share content with others who have similar interests. People who love country music are not forced to listen to hip-hop on MySpace; they can find other people who want to talk about Garth Brooks. If no one has started a group on a topic, they can be the first, and others can find them.

TIP

Web 2.0 gives nurses— and anyone else— the opportunity to contribute.

eBay is another great example. Think about how hard it is for someone interested in collecting, trading, and selling white, glazed-porcelain cats (or any other rare collectible) before the advent of the World Wide Web! There might not have been anyone in the collector's neighborhood, town, city, or even state who was interested in buying or trading. The Internet changed that, enabling the collector to create a web page and to buy, sell, and trade wares with fellow enthusiasts around the world.

Bringing Web 2.0 back to nursing, think about the last article you read online. Hopefully, it was useful. But even if it wasn't, odds are you were able to add your opinions, thoughts, or knowledge, or read other nurses' comments.

Table 1.1 compares traditional media, Web 1.0, and Web 2.0.

1.1 — Let's Compare

Traditional Media	Web 1.0	Web 2.0
Encyclopedia	Reference material	Wikipedia
Résumé or journal	Personal website	Blogging service
Address book	Guest book or directory	Facebook, LinkedIn
Tape or CD	mp3.com	MySpace
Mail	Evite	meetup.com
Videotapes, DVDs, movie store	N/A	YouTube, Vimeo, Hulu, Netflix
Collaborate by passing a single hard-copy document, created using a typewriter or word processor, from person to person	Collaborate by e-mailing a document to group members, one after the other	Collaborate using a shared online document that everyone can edit at the same time

If the Internet continues to grow, how do you keep up?

There are two basic ways to find and keep up to date with information: search and subscription.

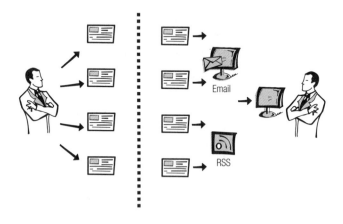

Figure 1.4: Search and subscription.

How does searching work?

In 2006, the verb "to Google" was added to the Oxford English Dictionary. As you probably know, the term refers to the use of the popular Internet search engine Google (Bylund, 2006). Although Google isn't the only search engine available—nor was it the first—the site's strength lies in its ability to find relevant information. Google achieves this by using an algorithm that takes into account the number of other pages that link to a given page in the search results. For example, people link to Wikipedia on a regular basis, which is why articles from that site often appear in the top 10 Google search results. Table 1.2 illustrates changes in the way people find information with Web 2.0.

1.2   Finding Information

Traditional	Web 1.0	Web 2.0
Ask someone you know.	Think of keywords and try searching domain names—for example, nurse.com, hospitalresources.com, or centralhospital.com.	Use a search engine for keywords: nursing, health care, etc.
Visit a library and ask the librarian for help, using index cards.		Search within websites for professional organizations, educational institutions, and governments—for example, Sigma Theta Tau International, FDA.
Check research journal and other expert sources.	Try to find a directory; go through all the links and hope they are up to date.	
	Search Geocities for people with similar interests who might have links to good websites.	Use a blog search engine such as blogsearch.google.com.

How do subscriptions work?

Once users find a relevant site, the challenge becomes how to stay up to date. One approach is to submit your name to a website's mailing list to receive periodic e-mails from the site. Another is to subscribe to the site's RSS feed, if it has one. Then, the RSS (short for Really Simply Syndication) feed will be delivered to the user's RSS feed reader automatically. This feed reader acts like a customized newspaper of sorts, compiling "article" feeds from all your favorite websites with the newest stories on the front page. This is much easier than manually entering URLs for 20 nursing-resource websites and browsing for new content!

TIP

You'll learn more about RSS later in this book.

Why has Web 2.0 been successful?

Web 2.0 has been successful for a number of reasons:

* Every user, or consumer, can also be a producer.
* Users can add links and connect websites themselves.
* Increased participation allows for coverage of niche interests.
* Participation facilitates rapid content growth.
* Search allows users to find more relevant information.
* Subscription services enable users to keep up with specific content.

What do nurses need to know about Web 2.0?

With Web 2.0, Internet users are transitioning from being passive consumers to active participants. Nurses must understand how patients use the Internet, as well as how they themselves use the Internet.

Becoming aware of popular and credible online resources for your patient population is a good start. Patients cannot always think of what questions they want to ask; when they get home, they may search for additional information about their condition. Along with any reference material your organization provides, consider whether there are online resources you can recommend.

As educated professionals with a wealth of knowledge from working in different clinical environments, nurses should feel empowered to participate online. In the past, a traditional approach to responding to newspaper articles was to write a letter to the editor. Now, users can share their opinions simply by submitting a comment. With professional resources, sharing your personal opinion is a valuable way to contribute your knowledge and experiences as they relate to what you are reading.

Insights & Inspiration

Daniel Gracie, RN

@hoyce

http://www.linkedin.com/in/danielgracie

With Web 2.0, nurses can create sites that discuss issues in their practice, participate in policy debates, engage in distance learning, and more easily share information with their colleagues. The easier access to information and ability to participate provide additional avenues for nurses to engage in and share professional communication and collaboration. Searching the Internet in the early days was not much better than going to a library for articles. With the evolution of Web 2.0, articles now come to us and we can receive practice questions from across the globe in no time. We as nurses can express ourselves among colleagues from our own organization or among peers across the globe.

Not only has the Internet changed, but also the tools it provides. I use many different sites for professional involvement and education. I can easily stay up to date with other nurses, nursing-related journals, accreditation groups, and nursing discussions online. I can send out a question and receive answers in a matter of minutes from around the world. Following nursing journals and scholarly groups allows me to preview or know about pertinent nursing articles the moment they are released, rather than waiting for them to arrive in the mail. Accreditation groups, such as The Joint Commission, often post bits of information providing further rationale behind their standards. This educational benefit has provided me with knowledge that frequently proves valuable at work and in school. Web 2.0 allows nurses the opportunity to do more than hunt and gather information.

Lesson: Look for ways you can participate on nursing websites, such as signing online petitions, completing surveys, or joining online discussions.

How has the Web evolved since the advent of Web 2.0?

When you read a book, there is no easy way to communicate with the author or with others reading the same book. With today's

World Wide Web, all that has changed. In addition to consuming content, users can produce it. They can also become aware of, and connect with, others who are consuming the same content (see Figure 1.5). Comments, user profiles, and social networks enable users to engage and collaborate in new ways.

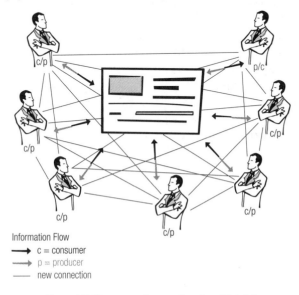

Figure 1.5: The power of connections from Web 2.0.

This development is what has made websites such as Facebook, LinkedIn, and Wikipedia really take off. In particular, Facebook has become popular, because it facilitates sharing personal information. It helps users contact each other and makes it easier to organize events. Users can share anything—from their hobbies to their experiences with cancer—and they do. Of course, some people feel that enabling others to learn more about them is a privacy issue. But Web 2.0 isn't about exposing personal secrets. It's about exposing information that users reveal and want to share.

TIP To better understand the potential of Web 2.0, watch Clay Shirky's 2009 TED talk: http://goo. gl/3L5MJ.

How are patients using the Internet?

According to the *Journal of Medical Internet Research,* more than half (68%) of adults report searching the Internet for health information, and patients with a chronic disease are affected by the information they find (Kreps, Beckjord, Atkinson, Saperstein, & Pleis, 2009). And findings by the Pew Internet and American Life Project show that 75% of patients who found health information online said it affected their decisions about treatment; 69% of patients made the decision to see a physician or get a second opinion based on their search results; and 57% of patients changed the way they manage their chronic disease (Fox, 2007). Clearly, health care providers need to develop the skills to participate online—for their own benefit, as well as their patients' sake.

Is there anything else you need to know about the Internet?

Unfortunately, a book such as this one can never fully convey every nuance of what is possible with the Internet. But Figure 1.6, which shows a "dummy" web page, should help you understand certain terms and references used throughout the book. You can use this "anatomy" of a web page as a cheat sheet.

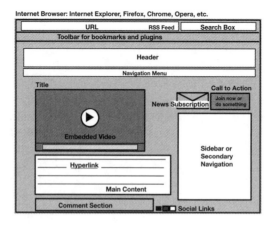

Figure 1.6: The "anatomy" of a Web page.

* URL—Uniform Resource Locator is a technical way to say a unique way to identify each web page. Entering a URL in the address bar will bring you to the website you wish to visit, such as http://pubmed.com.

* Toolbar—Menus and buttons that give additional functionality to the web browser, such as easy access to your bookmarks or a way to save a picture of the website.

* Search box—Due to the popularity of using a search engine to find a website, web browsers often include a search box, so you can start a search without first going to the search engine's web page.

* Header—Space at the top of a website that is often used for a logo or branding information. It may have a navigation bar as well.

* RSS feed—RSS feed logos will often be presented in the web browser address bar to allow you to easily identify the opportunity to subscribe to updates.

* Title—The heading at the beginning of an article or new section of content.

* News subscription—Many websites offer subscription options for users to receive updates, to keep visitors returning to the website.

* Call to action—Websites are created for different purposes. To accomplish goals, icons or buttons often request that visitors do something—for example, buy a product, complete a survey, or sign a petition.

* Navigation menu—Provides users easy access to information and helps visitors understand how a website is organized.

* Sidebar or secondary navigation—Offers additional options for accessing different pieces of information at a deeper level than the main navigation menu.

* Embedded content—Rich content such as video, pictures, and audio can be placed within the content, so you don't have to download the file.

* Hyperlinks—Using hyperlinks, authors can reference other web pages, making it easier for visitors to access additional content for more information.

* Main content—Provides the major content of interest on a particular web page.

* Comment section—Located below many content sections, this section offers the opportunity to comment. Visitors can see what others think of the content.

* Social links—Placing icons of commonly used social media tools on the page encourages users to save, share, or comment on the content.

Exploring Social Media

How are patients using social media?

No patient or hospital is the same, but there are some great examples of how patients and providers are starting to use the new tools available to them. Patients Like Me (www.patientslikeme.com) is one of those examples of patients and providers using social media. Because Facebook is not the right space for discussing disease symptoms, Patients Like Me—PLM for short—was started to enable users to share their disease history. This online resource doesn't try to tell patients what having epilepsy or Parkinson's disease is like. Instead, PLM enables users to share data on more than 20 diseases and develop meaningful relationships with other patients and with care providers who join the network.

How are nurses using social media?

Searching the Internet for keywords such as nurse and blog, or running a search for nurse on social media sites such as Twitter, Facebook, and LinkedIn, quickly reveals that nurses are using social media. However, consistency in how nurses use social media is lacking. Hopefully, by the time you finish reading this book, you will have clear ideas about how you can use social media to advance your career.

How can you tell if you're on a social media site?

To determine whether a website supports the use of social media, consider whether the site allows you to easily share content and whether any of its content is user—generated. Look for the elements shown in Table 1.3.

1.3 Commonly Used Social Media Symbols and Icons

Image or Logo	Meaning	Purpose
	E-mail and RSS	Easily subscribe to content
LEAVE A COMMENT	Comment section	Contribute ideas or comments
	Social network logos	Easily send links to friends or professional contacts who might enjoy the content
delicious / diigo	Bookmarking tools	Easily bookmark page to find it later
facebook	Sign up or join	Create a profile to give others additional information about yourself, if they are interested.

Exercises

Now that you understand how the Internet has evolved, let's do a bit of sightseeing on the World Wide Web.

1. Open your computer's web browser and go to the websites of nursing organizations in your state or province—for example, the website for your local union, professional association, or regulatory body. If you know a site's URL, enter it directly in your web browser's address bar. Alternatively, use Google (http://www.google.com) or Bing (http://www.bing.com) to find the site. If you can't think of any sites to visit, go to http://rnao.org or http://www.icn.ch/. Then visit http://mayoclinic.com and http://engadget.com. As you visit these sites, consider the following:

   * How easy is each site to use?

   * Which website is more engaging? Which is easiest to navigate?

   * Can you easily provide comments or subscribe to newsletters?

   * How does the site provide information—text only, text with pictures, or video?

   * Are there icons and links to social networking sites, such as Facebook and Twitter, so you can share articles with friends?

2. Now go to your favorite search engine and type in some keywords related to your interests in nursing. Next, use the same search terms in http://blogsearch.google.com and http://twitter.com. Are you able to find something interesting? If so, click on the links to three websites and evaluate those sites using the same criteria as before.

3. Think about topics that you feel more people (nurses, nursing students, patients, etc.) need to know about. Do you have ideas or content you want to share with others? If you didn't have to do the "techy" stuff, what type of website would you want to be in charge of?

2

*

Understanding the Basic Building Blocks of Social Media

Do you:

Think all websites are the same?

Get confused when thinking about websites and online tools?

Feel nervous when someone asks if they can "friend" you?

Know that "Facebook" and "tweet" are verbs as well as nouns?

Understand the basic categories of social media tools?

Imagine a drawer, stuffed to the brim with tools. These could be any type of tools—makeup accessories, stationery, cleaning products, construction tools, whatever. When you pull open that messy drawer, with tools spilling out all over the place, can you easily identify and locate everything? No. When you look at a disorganized mess, it is hard to understand what each tool is used for.

This chapter provides ways to think about, assess, categorize, and understand the most common Internet and social media tools. The more you understand how to use social media services, the more you can learn about what matters most to your work—and the easier it will be to use these tools to help your career.

Note that the tools cited in this chapter do not comprise a complete list of those available. The Internet is ever-expanding, growing as new tools are created.

Understanding the Differences

Is every website the same?

No. Just as every person is different, every website is different. Even if two websites seem similar, they may have very different tools and require different skill sets. Think about nurses. All nurses are similar at some level, but does that mean you can put pediatric nurses in an adult emergency room? Not if you want them to be effective.

The first chapter discussed how the Internet has changed. This is similar to talking about how transportation has changed from human- and animal-powered vehicles to ones that run on gasoline and jet fuel. This chapter discusses how websites can be both similar and different, as a public bus is both similar to and different from a bullet train.

How are sites different?

A web page is a simply a document. Groups of web pages make up a website. Generally, websites are developed for two reasons. The first is to share information with a specific audience. The second is to enable visitors to perform certain activities. These two categories are defined as follows:

* Content—Content websites focus on specific topics and subjects, and may use different tools to share information.

* Services—These websites perform a function and can be used for different subjects or topics.

Content websites include news sites or topic-specific sites such as the Sigma Theta Tau International website (http://www.nursingsociety.org). Content-driven sites focus on a specific audience and vary their method of information delivery. Service sites are more general sites such as Google (http://www.google.com), which allow individuals to use the service to meet their own needs. Knowing the difference between a content-focused site and a service-oriented site will help you grasp how to best utilize the website.

How do you evaluate a website?

You can apply the nursing process (assess, diagnose, plan, do, evaluate) to critically think about websites:

* Assess

* Is this website focused on content or service?

* Content—Is the content credible, reliable, useful, or interesting?

* Service—What does this service do? Would this be useful for you? How could you use this service—with friends and family (personal)? Or to learn, research, or share information related to work (professional)?

* Diagnose

* This website is a content/service website that (focuses on/ allows me to) _____.

* This website is or is not good at____.

* This website is or is not very useful to me.

* Plan

* I should come back to this website if I want to find information about _____ (content) or when I want to do _____ (service).

* I know that _____ might find this (useful or interesting); I should share it with him or her.

* Do

* Do what you plan.

* Evaluate

* This website is good for what I want to do.

* This website is not good for what I want to do. I should find another one.

What other information can you use to assess websites?

Both content- and service-based websites are becoming more integrated. For example, content sites now have services built in, such as search functionality or profiles for frequent users. The same can be said for service-oriented sites. For example, websites that host videos, such as YouTube, have users who upload content on specific topics, such as nursing. Understanding this integration can make sites more useful. If you are on a content-focused website, look for services the site might support. If you visit a service website, explore to see whether it hosts any content that interests you.

TIP

Social media sites are great ways to share knowledge, as well as find it.

Content-based websites make sense, but what service websites are available?

There are many different types of web services, and the number keeps growing. More often than not, these services have multiple capabilities. Some are good for helping you get in touch with old friends. Others help you find different forms of information.

How do you categorize web tools?

Frankly, the sheer number of tools on the Web is intimidating. But once you start to understand what each tool was designed to do, you can begin to mentally organize them. To do this, you need to be familiar with some of the commonly used tools and understand the primary function of each one. This will help you start to make sense of the complexity.

"Technologies which have had the most profound effect on human life are usually simple."

–Freeman Dyson

Messaging

What is messaging?

During the early stages of the Internet, one of the first services offered was messaging. Examples of messaging include electronic mail (e-mail) and instant messaging (IM). These online tools can greatly reduce the cost of communication. They may not replicate the thought and intent that can be put into a personalized birthday card, but they do lower the barrier for a lot of communication.

What is e-mail?

As you no doubt know, e-mail enables users to send messages (text) and attachments (computer files) to other individuals or multiple people. It's the online version of mail. E-mail is great for business and personal correspondence. It provides an easy mode of contact as well as a single place to collect and respond to messages. Examples of free e-mail services include Gmail (http://gmail.com), Yahoo! Mail (http://www.yahoo.com/mail), and AOL Mail (http://www.mail.aol.com).

What does e-mail enable you to do?

With e-mail, you can

* Send and receive e-mail messages

* Organize e-mail messages into folders for easy retrieval

* Locate messages using a search function

* Store e-mails

E-mail is a great option for personal correspondence. Filtering helps you manage your inbox, so important e-mails don't get buried. Plus, e-mail services offer a large amount of storage, meaning you can archive old e-mails rather than delete them.

What is instant messaging?

With instant messaging, you can have real-time "chat" sessions—that is, text-based conversations online. It represents a cheap and easy way to have conversations while in different locations, and you can often use both voice and video chat. Examples of instant messaging services include Google Talk (http://www.google.com/talk), AOL Instant Messenger (http://www.aim.com), Windows Live Messenger (http://messenger.msn.com), and Skype (http://skype.com).

What can you do with instant messaging?

With instant messaging, you can

* See when contacts are online and available to chat

* Change your status when you're online; options include available, away, and appear offline

* Have real-time, text-based conversations with friends, family, and professional contacts online

* Share computer files with contacts

With instant messaging, you can contact friends or family. You can see when they are available by checking their status. You can also ask for help or information from a contact who is online.

"The first ten years of the Internet revolution were all about getting computers connected to the World Wide Web. But the next ten years are going to be all about getting people connected to each other."

–Dave McClure

Social Networking

What is social networking?

One of the most popular Internet tools is social networking. Using social networks is an easy way to keep up with friends and family, and share information and current events widely. Social networks can also be used to develop relationships with people you may not see or interact with as often.

These sites are directories that provide additional information about individuals and offer services to share information and content and communicate with others on the social networking site. There are two types:

Personal networking sites—Using this type of site, you can create a personal profile, connect with other users, and share meaningful information (messages, pictures, videos, etc.). Facebook (http://www.facebook.com) is the largest of these sites. With more than 500 million users (and growing), Facebook makes it easy to find people you know. The site is renowned for providing simple tools for building a personal profile, numerous ways to share content and organize events and groups, and integration with many outside websites. Other options (though significantly less popular) include Bebo (http://bebo.com) and Hi5 (http://www.Hi5.com).

Professional networking sites—With this type of site, you can create a professional profile and connect with other professional individuals, groups, or organizations. Profiles and services are focused around work; you enter your work history, education, research interest, special skills, and awards and share this information with others. Participating in these networks makes it easier for you to manage your contacts, stay up to date with your contacts' job transitions, and make yourself available to those seeking your expertise. LinkedIn (http://www.linkedin.com) is one of the largest professional networks; it enables you to create a profile that resembles a résumé. You can also use the site to create professional groups and organizational profiles. Another option—though considerably less popular—is Mendeley (http://www.mendeley.com).

What can you do on a personal social networking site?

With personal social networking sites, such as Facebook, you can

* Easily customize your profile with personal information, such as interests, hobbies, music preferences, pictures, etc.

* "Friend" other users—that is, request to connect with them on the social network site and have them agree (or vice versa); you can then view and post messages on each other's profiles

* Upload pictures and videos easily

* Create groups to organize friends around causes or interests, or use fan pages to create a professional profile for your organization, business, or cause

How can personal social networking sites help nurses?

Nurses can use personal social networking sites to

* Stay in touch with family and friends

* Develop friendships with colleagues

* Support and promote causes, events, and organizations

* Connect with others with shared interests or hobbies

What can you do on a professional social networking site?

Using a professional social networking site, such as LinkedIn or Sigma Theta Tau International's The Circle (http://thecircle. nursingsociety.org/), you can

* Easily enter professional experience and skills

* Participate in groups with shared professional interests—for example, the Hospital Infection Control group

* Manage your professional contacts without fear of the information becoming outdated when colleagues change jobs

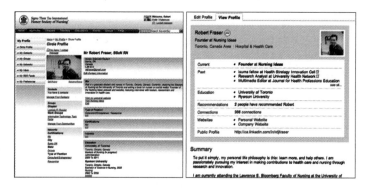

Figure 2.1: With professional networking sites such as The Circle and LinkedIn, you can highlght your professional interests, experience, and knowledge.

How can professional social networking sites help nurses?

Nurses can use professional social networking sites to

* Share their work history with others

* Find other nurses with similar work interests and specialties

* Stay in touch with people met at work functions, conferences, or on the job

Content Sharing

What is content sharing?

This category refers to the various types of media (audio, video, and pictures) and document files (word-processing documents, Power-Point presentations, and PDF files) that can be shared on the Web. More and more, people want to access these files while surfing the Internet and share them with their social networks.

What is video sharing?

With video sharing, users—whether individuals or companies—can watch videos online and upload their videos to share, without having to pay for website hosting or traffic costs. The most popular video-sharing site is YouTube (http://www.youtube.com), which enables users to post video clips up to 10 minutes long (or longer, if users apply for special permission). Other examples of video-sharing websites are Vimeo (http://vimeo.com) and Blip.tv (http://www.blip.tv).

What can you do on a video-sharing site?

By using video-sharing sites, such as YouTube, you can

* Upload video content for free

* Create a channel for posting certain types of content

* Take video from YouTube and embed it into your own website

* Read other users' profiles and subscribe to users who regularly post content of interest to you (in this way, YouTube is a type of social networking site)

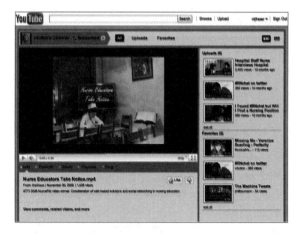

Figure 2.2: Nurses with all types of interests can share videos they have made. Vernon Dutton has an avid interest in nursing history.

How can video-sharing sites help nurses?

Nurses can use video-sharing sites to

* Demonstrate health tips (for example, hand hygiene) or to educate patients

* Find instructional videos for learning

* Upload interviews or speeches

What is audio sharing?

With audio sharing, users can upload audio files to share with others and find recordings on topics in which they are interested. This alternative to text-based sharing is helpful for certain types of information or for users who are visually impaired. One example of an audio-sharing website is PodoMatic (http://podomatic.com), which provides free audio hosting for a limited number of files and a method for submitting new files to directories. Another option is Blog Talk Radio (http://www.blogtalkradio.com).

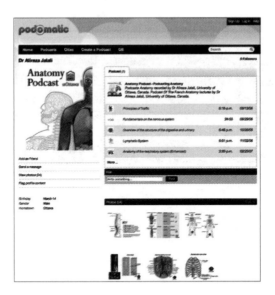

Figure 2.3: You can upload audio, video, and images to PodoMatic to share information with others. Dr. Alireza Jalali uses it to upload lectures from the University of Ottawa.

What can you do on an audio-sharing site?

With audio-sharing sites, such as PodoMatic, you can

* Upload audio recordings of lectures, interviews, or conference presentations

* Create a podcast—that is, an audio series on a certain topic that users can listen to online or download to a computer or portable listening device

How can audio-sharing sites help nurses?

Nurses can use audio-sharing sites to

* Create regular radio-style shows that discuss specific topics, such as emergency nursing or nursing news

* Share lectures or talks with a wider audience than may be able to attend events in person

What is picture sharing?

With picture sharing, users can share and browse pictures online. This is much easier than sharing a real-life photo album or mailing pictures to family and friends. The largest and most popular photo-sharing service, Flickr (http://www.flickr.com), enables users to upload high-quality images and to set copyrights to restrict or allow others to use images as they desire. Picasa, another picture-sharing site (http://www.picasa.com), is owned by Google.

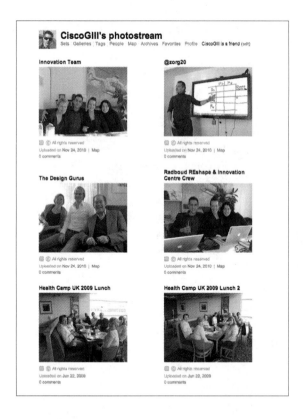

Figure 2.4: Flickr is a great photo-sharing site that can be used to share all sorts of images. Francisco Grajales used Flickr to share pictures from his trips to Europe for health care conferences and research meetings.

What can you do on a picture-sharing site?

With picture-sharing sites, such as Flickr, you can

* Upload images and organize them into albums

* Tag images with keywords, so users can search for pictures

How can picture-sharing sites help nurses?

Nurses can use picture-sharing sites to

* Upload and share images from conferences that might be useful for others

* Find images to use in a presentation

What is a document repository?

With a document repository, users can upload presentations and documents and embed them in their websites. As presentations and reports become more common, using document-sharing sites such as these will help you to get a better return from the effort you put into your work. One popular document repository, SlideShare (http:// slideshare.net), specializes in sharing PowerPoint documents. Users can even do voiceovers on their slides and can also upload other types of documents to the site. Scribd (http://scribd.com) is another example of a document repository.

What can you do on a document repository?

With document-repository sites, such as SlideShare, you can

* Upload presentations and view PowerPoint presentations on-line

* Embed content in other websites

* Allow other users to find your work during searches

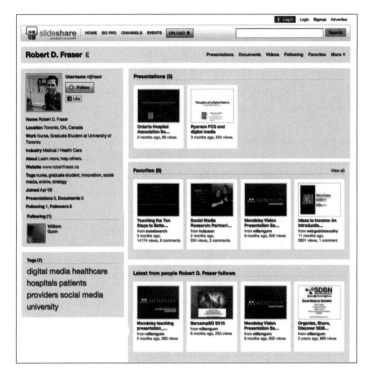

Figure 2.5: Sharing presentations you prepared for a conference, lecture, or seminar is easy using SlideShare.

How can document repositories help nurses?

Nurses can use document repositories to

* Repurpose work they have done for school or work to help others learn

* Find experts on topics they are interested in and learn from their presentations

Web Publishing

What is web publishing?

Very few nurses are full-time authors or researchers, meaning we do not spend most of our time writing and publishing our ideas. However, that does not mean our ideas cannot add value to our professional knowledge and the public's knowledge. The opportunities to publish information online are increasing. With web publishing, you can publish content online without having to learn the complex languages of the Internet. There are services that let you regularly post articles and organize them by date (blogs), design and build your own websites (customizable web pages), and even publish short updates about what you are doing (microblogging). Many of these services are free and can serve as useful tools for nurses.

"Publishing your work is important. Even if you are giving a piece to some smaller publication for free, you will learn something about your writing. The editor will say something, friends will mention it. You will learn."

—Tim Cahill

What is blogging?

Blogging enables users to post content online on a special page called a blog, short for web log. Blog entries, called posts, are organized by time, with the most recent post being featured at the top of the web page hosting the blog. More sophisticated blogs also have categories to help users find posts of interest, rather than simply what is new.

A blog is a simple way for individuals to publish information online that is important or interesting to them. Blogs can vary widely in use, which is one reason they are so powerful. Users can develop content over time. As bloggers talk more about their topic, other sites may begin to link to their articles. As a result, the blog will appear higher in the list of results in search engines. WordPress (http://wordpress.com), one popular blogging service, is highly customizable and boasts additional functions for organizing content. Other options include Tumblr (http://tumblr.com) and Posterous (http://posterous.com).

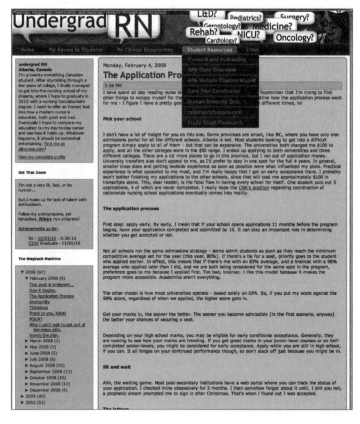

Figure 2.6: Even nursing students can use blogs to share information such as advice on nursing school applications and useful study resources. UndergradRN (http://undergradrn.blogspot.com) is a great example of how nurses can use a blog.

What can you do on a blog?

With blogging, you can

* Publish content

* Embed files such as videos and pictures directly in blog posts

* Organize posts into categories to allow viewers to better find content, similar to how books are divided into chapters and magazines are separated into sections

* Tag posts and pages to help visitors find coverage of topics they are interested in, similar to how a book index works

How can blogging help nurses?

Nurses can use blogging to

* Reflect on practice or professional experience and learn from each other

* Share expertise on a topic such as public health or emergency nursing

* Share links to their favorite online resources

What is a customizable web page?

Using customizable web pages, you can quickly and easily create a simple website to share any information you choose, without having to learn a programming language such as HTML (or pay someone to create the page for you). One site that enables users to build customizable web pages is Google Sites (http://sites.google.com). Google Sites provides pre-designed site and page templates, as well as tools for editing content and controlling access to the site. Webs (http://webs.com) is another site where you can create a customizable web page.

What can you do on a customizable web page?

With a customizable web page, you can

* Skip the design stage, because the templates are pre-designed; simply enter the information you want to share in the desired area of the page

* Include pictures, videos, and other files on web pages

How can customizable web pages help nurses?

Nurses can use customizable web pages to

* Build a professional portfolio or personal website highlighting their skills or business services

* Promote clubs or professional activities

* Educate other nurses or staff

* Share details about projects or research

What is microblogging?

Microblogs let users share very small (micro) amounts of information, arranging that information in chronological order, similar to a blog. Microblogging has become popular because it provides an easy way to update others without sending each person a message or spending a lot of time writing. Thanks to the development of mobile apps—that is, microblogging applications that you can use on the go via a smart phone—users can share what they are doing as they do it, whether it is reading an interesting article or watching a news story unfold.

The most popular microblogging service is Twitter (http://twitter. com). Using Twitter, users can post updates, or tweets, containing no more than 140 characters (letters and spaces). Twitter is famous for breaking news stories before the traditional news stations can—and, of course, for posts on what people are eating for lunch. Another example of a microblogging site is Yammer (http://yammer. com).

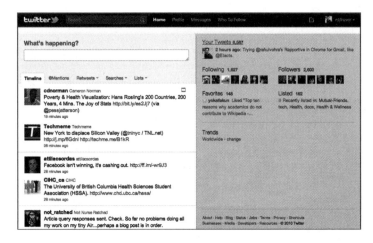

Figure 2.7: Updates are pulled into your Twitter stream, so you can easily follow what people are doing.

What can you do with a microblog?

With a microblog, you can

* Easily sign up and begin sharing information

* Use these very simple services to share and interact with others

* Create a news feed (on Twitter, called a Twitter stream) that pulls in updates from selected users that you have chosen to follow

* Follow friends, news sources, colleagues, and thought leaders online

How can microblogging help nurses?

Nurses can use microblogging to

* Share information with others, such as journal articles, news updates, and other important information

* Share expertise

* Develop a personal and professional reputation

* Create a filtered news source to help them find content of interest

Collaborating

How can you collaborate using social media?

Social media tools don't just provide a way to develop content and share information; they also make it possible for individuals and groups to work together. Anyone who has ever edited a paper or tried to put together a group presentation knows that determining who has the most up-to-date document or the current state of the project can be very challenging. Collaborative tools, such as document-editing tools and wikis, help users work together at different times and in different places on the same project.

What are document-editing tools?

Document-editing tools make it possible for more than one person to access and edit documents of various types, including spreadsheets, text documents, and PowerPoint presentations. Using these tools, users can edit documents from any computer connected to the Internet and share work with others in real time to finish a project more quickly. Google Docs (http://docs.google.com) is one type of document-editing tool. With this tool, users can work on documents, spreadsheets, presentations, drawings, and surveys—all at the same time, from different locations. Another document-sharing tool is Docs.com (http://docs.com).

TIP

Learning is never finished, whether it centers on social media tools or updating your understanding of clinical practice.

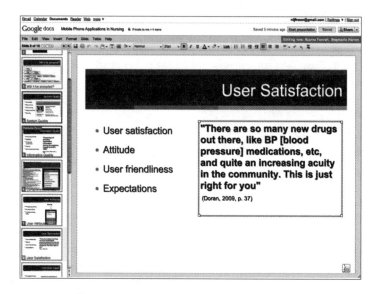

Figure 2.8: Google Docs is useful for preparing assignments, finishing reports, and completing presentations with colleagues and coworkers.

What can you do with document-editing tools?

With document-editing tools, you can

* Access a shared document at your convenience

* Edit a document at the same time as another user

* Keep the document up to date, which means you don't have to worry that someone else has a newer version of the document

How can document-editing tools help nurses?

Nurses can use document-editing tools to

* Work on school assignments or unit projects

* Share documents such as schedules or policies with other users; the ability to edit the document can be turned off in these instances

* Collaborate with others in different cities and countries

What are wikis?

Wikis are online collaborative websites where users can add new pages and edit existing ones. Working in groups online can be difficult; often, coordinating a project or sharing knowledge is not easy to do online. With wikis, groups can easily share information and, most importantly, edit and update that information as each member contributes and the project evolves. Wikipedia (http://wikipedia.org) is one well-known example of a wiki. On Wikipedia, anyone can edit an online encyclopedia using wiki technology. Other examples are Wikispaces (http://wikispaces.com), where users can sign up to create their own public or private wiki for collaboration with others, and PBworks (http://pbworks.com).

What can you do with a wiki?

With wikis, you can

* Quickly and easily add new users

* Make the space private and protect it with a password

* Create new pages and share resources

* Find older versions of information in case of accidental deletion

How can wikis help nurses?

Nurses can use wikis to

* Work on hospital projects, such as creating unit policies and guidelines

* Share information and keep it up to date

* Organize projects or events

* Work with a group on multiple documents with different types of information

Frequently Asked Questions

 How can you possibly remember all of these tools?

You can't. Although the mind has an incredible capacity to learn new information, it cannot retain everything at once. Think about all the signs you have to memorize when learning to drive a car, or how much knowledge you have picked up in school and on the job as a nurse. There is no way you could have learned all that in one sitting. If reading about these tools simply results in one or two moments of inspiration, that is perfect. It's like learning anatomy: You start by understanding how one or two pieces work, and soon everything begins to fit together. Understanding these building blocks doesn't mean you'll know how to use every tool, and that's OK. As you read this book, simply remember what tools you are using and how they might work well with others. Recognizing what you can do with a tool will not only give you insight in how to use it, it will also help you recognize how to transfer skills to other web services.

 What is the best way to start?

There are three ways to begin. First, if you see someone using an online tool that you might want to use yourself, simply replicate that use. Second, experiment. If you have an idea for how a tool might be used, try it. Finally, if you know other people who are using an online tool that you do not understand, explore the technology. Maybe you'll find the tool to be useful, or maybe you won't. But even if you find that the tool will not help you with what you are currently working on, knowing what tools are out there may come in handy in the future.

 Is Facebook better than LinkedIn?

Better is a very subjective word. Facebook is primarily for personal relationships and for interests that focus around social connections. LinkedIn is clearly the professional-driven network. If you are looking to manage your business contacts and would like for others to approach you with job opportunities or collaboration ideas, then a professional network such as LinkedIn is probably the way to go. But, using Facebook to keep in touch with old classmates or friends from work in a social manner can be just as useful. Each tool offers its advantages; creating your own profile and learning how these tools work are probably the best ways to understand what is best for you.

 ## What are the differences among the various blogging services?

Choosing among social media tools (social networks, blogs, etc.) is like choosing among a car, truck, or boat. Each has its own specialty. Choosing among different tools that offer the same basic service—such as whether to start your blog on Wordpress or Tumblr—is similar to choosing between Ford and Dodge trucks. Each service differs in its features, strengths, and weaknesses. You may have to test drive a few to find the right fit. Another option is to learn from others' experience. For example, you might take a look at other blogs you like and then use the same blogging service. If you cannot find examples to follow, do some more research. Think about what features you like best, and then try a service for yourself.

 ## How often do you have to use these sites?

Remember, these sites are now your free tools. How you use them is up to you. Take the analogy of a hammer: A carpenter will likely use her hammer on a daily basis, but a hobbyist might use his only occasionally. Compare this to a blog. Depending on how you use your blog, you might post your favorite research papers quarterly, or you could post something every day for a week when you are inspired—for example, to share tips with new nurses. As you learn how you want to utilize web services, the answer to this question will become more clear.

Exercises

1. Instead of simply reading a book on social media, watch a few short videos. To begin, open your Internet browser and go to http://youtube.com. Once there, search for "social networking in plain English" to find a short video on social networks.

2. Run a new search on YouTube to find a video about a different social media tool you are curious about. If you can't think of any, try searching for "using SlideShare"; then pick a video or two to watch.

3. Look for some presentations on social media tools. To begin, go to http://slideshare.net; then use the site's search tools to find a presentation on social media. For example, try searching for "learning to use social media." Look at a few presentations and see what you can learn.

4. Run a new search on SlideShare for "12 leads made easy" or "learning ECG" and look at some of the presentations available on these topics. The point isn't to learn about these topics; rather, it's to get you thinking about how to find information you are interested in or how you could present information you know.

3

*

Privacy, Disclaimers, and Professional Issues

Do you:

Understand the professional standards you are accountable to?

Think you could be fired for having a blog?

Know what filters you need to consider when posting online?

Know what good standards for using social media are?

Know what information you should disclose on your website?

As discussed in previous chapters, social media is a powerful tool that can spread information more quickly and to a wider audience than was ever possible before. But, when using social media, every nurse must be aware of the potential risks.

Think of social media as being a tool, just like a needle. A needle cannot tell whether it is administering a safe amount of medication or if it is being used in the right way. Similar to using a needle, nurses using social media must understand the risks and how to prevent adverse events. To safely use social media, it's essential that you understand your professional responsibilities.

Professionalism

Who is responsible for your actions?

As a nurse, you are a licensed health care professional. With that title comes responsibility. When acting as a nurse, you are ultimately responsible for your actions. Whether you are riding a bus home with a colleague, administering a needle, or sending a letter to a newspaper, you must always think critically about your legal and professional responsibilities. A simple conversation overheard can violate patient confidentiality; not understanding safe practices can harm patients; and an inappropriate letter printed in the newspaper can have professional re-percussions. Going online is no different—it only magnifies your audience. You must think critically about your actions and consider your professional filters to determine what is appropriate.

TIP

Take responsibility for all your actions online.

What are professional filters?

Professional filters are barriers set in place to prevent harm and maximize positive results. Professional filters include the following (see Figure 3.1):

* Government—Government creates laws that nurses must follow or face financial or criminal penalties.

* Nursing regulators—These national and regional bodies control who is fit to practice as a nurse, set standards for nurses, and decide when individuals have failed to met these standards. Punishment from your regulatory body can include suspension or revocation of your nursing license.

✴ Employers—Employers set rules and policies for how employees should act at work and how employees can or cannot represent the company. Companies have the right to discipline and possibly terminate employment if individuals fail to follow the organizational policy.

✴ Professional standards—These are set by professional associations and act as ideal guidelines. These guidelines help nurses identify the best way to deal with issues. If they are not followed, it simply means that the ideal did not occur; it does not imply any wrongdoing.

✴ Personal judgment—This final filter influences an individual's actions.

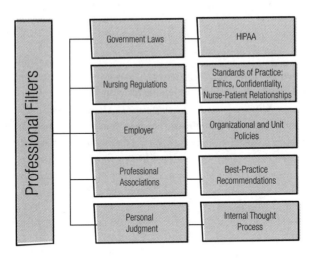

Figure 3.1: Illustration of the different filters nurses should apply when thinking about privacy.

Laws Pertaining to Social Media

What specific laws do you need to be aware of?

Nurses need to be aware of the Health Insurance Portability and Accountability Act (HIPAA), which protects patient confidentiality (Ressler & Glazer, 2010). In a nutshell, HIPAA makes it illegal to share any information about a particular person's health status, care provided to them, or how it was paid for beyond the expressed clinical use at your organization. This is why posting photographs, descriptions, or details that include patients is not recommended.

> *"Trust is the easiest thing in the world to lose and the hardest thing in the world to get back."*
>
> –R. Williams

The other laws that are important to consider are those pertaining to libel. These are designed to enable an individual to protect his or her image. Libel laws hold individuals responsible for false, malicious, or undeserved statements that hurt the reputation of an individual or a business (Givens, 2009). The key part to remember is that statements are only considered libel if they are not true or cannot be proven. Therefore, you must be very sure of the facts before posting information, especially if it could damage the reputation of a person or business.

How can you avoid breaking these laws?

Patient confidentiality and privacy are commonly discussed topics in health care. Consider how you would discuss work with family members or friends. Here are some tips to remember (see Table 3.1 for more information):

* Never use patient names or identifiers (phone numbers, hospital IDs, etc.)—Simply leaving out a last name, such as saying "My patient Bill," is not nearly good enough. Use a pseudonym and change irrelevant identifiers.

* Speak about patients in generalities—Discussing your experiences with challenging patients, nurse-physician relationships, and administration of medication is best done without referring to specific clients. Draw from multiple experiences without using details of one event.

* Do not disclose dates or time frames—Avoid posting comments that include words such as "today," "yesterday," or "last week." This type of information can be used to help identify a patient. Instead, use terms such as "recently," "in the past," or "over the years."

* Avoid discussing treatment location—Linking patient stories to a specific hospital or unit makes it easier to identify the patient. Even if it does not give away patient details, negatively discussing patients creates suspicion and distrust of nurses by the public. Would you want to be served at a bank where a teller was discussing how dumb customers were or how little money they had?

* Leaving out a single significant detail is not enough—Omitting a single piece of information is not enough if there are unique details around it. Remove and change as much information as possible.

TIP

Talk about general lessons learned, not specific patient experiences.

* Do not post pictures of patients—If a picture is worth a thousand words, just imagine how much information you're giving someone who recognizes details from a photograph.

Protect Yourself When You Post

Advice	Inappropriate Example	Appropriate Example
Never use patient identifiers.	"Working with Bill, an Army war veteran, I learned ..."	"Working with war veterans has taught me ..."
Speak in generalities, not specifics.	"Recently, a patient was admitted with a myocardial infarction, diabetes mellitus, and ..."	"Seeing patients with multiple health problems ..."
Do not disclose dates or time frames.	"Last month, my patient ..." "This week, I took care of ..." "Two years ago ..."	"I have had patients ..." "Over the years ..." "Previously ..."
Avoid discussing treatment location.	"Working in the ICU ..." "Patients in the emergency mental unit ..."	"In my experience ..." "Working in mental health ..."
Change or omit as many details as possible.	"Mrs. X's two daughters, who visited her when she was being treated for malignant carcinoma, could not accept the diagnosis and argued constantly with me and with the physician."	"Dealing with a patient's family members who are struggling to cope with a diagnosis can be challenging for nurses and physicians."
Do not post pictures of patients.	Caption: "Look at this leg ulcer! Amazing what can happen to the body."	DON'T DO IT.

Here are some strategies to help you avoid charges of libel (Givens, 2009):

* Avoid posting negative comments or opinions that you are unable to prove with facts. If you are charged with libel, it is your responsibility to prove that your statement is true.

* Posting statements that might damage an organization's or person's reputation is neither helpful nor a good practice. If you have an issue, the best approach is to deal directly with the individual or organization in question.

* Remember the saying "If you don't have anything nice to say, don't say anything at all." Posting negative comments about a person or a business does not fix the problem—and if they are untrue, it could be costly to you.

What if you use an anonymous account?

Choosing to share professional comments and opinions online and taking the extra step of obscuring your identify is not wrong. Many nurses and doctors prefer to use pseudonyms and fake identities. However, O'Reilly (2010) warns that anonymity may make it easier to act in ways that undermine public trust in health care professionals. In addition, it does not offer you protection if someone connects you to your online material. You will still be subject to prosecution if you commit libel or violate HIPAA if you are identified. Besides, if you are using social media to build your professional credibility or publicize your expertise, submitting content anonymously will not help you or your career.

Insights & Inspiration

Toronto Emergency Nurse

@torontoemerg

http://torontoemerg.wordpress.com

I started my blog in homage to the sometimes very funny and cynical physician and nurse bloggers who write about their experiences in health care. I'm an emergency nurse, after all: I had stories, and then some. I would write anonymously to protect the confidentiality of my patients, not to mention myself, and to give myself the freedom to write what I pleased. I would out-snark them all. So I tried sardonic and sarcastic. Trouble is, if you take writing seriously, bitter, angry, and hostile are not viable poses for the long haul. I began to wonder, too, if telling stories in this light reflected more on me as a nurse than on the putative silliness of my patients. And to be honest, cynical health care blogs are as common as cold days in a Toronto winter.

In any case, the stories start sounding the same after a while. Stupid is as stupid does. How many times could I write about some drunk guy being an idiot? If I was getting bored, what about my readers? So my voice changed, matured (I think), and became more reflective. I began to focus more on the power of nursing as a profession, and in our ability to articulate and critically evaluate important issues related to health care. The funny stories are still there, but much kinder. But I think my blog is better for the change, and frankly, my hits are way up since.

Lesson: Do not underestimate the power of social media; there is a lot more to it than trivial distractions like Farmville and Justin Bieber's Twitter updates. Using a blog or Twitter account can be a great way to cross-pollinate ideas between health care professionals working in all sorts of settings. These tools can also be used to make contact and create conversation between formal and informal leaders.

"Don't say anything online that you wouldn't want plastered on a billboard with your face on it."

–Erin Bury

Professional Regulations Pertaining to Social Media

What professional regulations do you need to be aware of?

Unfortunately, nursing organizations have not yet released policies on social media. However, the concerns that regulatory bodies most frequently mention include patient confidentiality, privacy, nurse-patient relationships, and codes of professional conduct.

Nurses can also learn from other professional organizations, such as the American Medical Association, which recommends that providers consider the following (Council on Ethical and Judicial Affairs, 2010):

* Be aware of privacy standards and patient confidentiality, which must be maintained at all times, including online.

* Privacy settings should be used to protect information when possible, but they are not an absolute security measure. Providers should realize that once on the Internet, information is no longer fully in your control and may be permanent. Therefore, providers should regularly monitor their own online accounts, websites, and information to ensure that content anyone posts is accurate and appropriate.

* If interacting with patients online, providers must maintain appropriate relationships according to professional and ethical standards.

* Providers should consider creating professional boundaries to separate personal and professional content online.

* Upon witnessing content posted by colleagues that appears unprofessional, providers have a responsibility to bring it to the attention of the individual, so he or she can take appropriate steps to remove it or initiate appropriate actions. If the behavior that violates professional standards or codes of conduct is not dealt with, the appropriate authorities should be informed.

What organizational policies do you need to adhere too?

The answer to this question depends on where you work. Ask your employer if the organization has a policy on or related to social media. Not every organization will have one, but such policies are becoming more common. If your organization has a policy, you are required to abide by it when at work or representing your organization.

If your organization bans the use of social media at work, what guidelines should you follow?

If your organization does not allow you to use social media while at work, that is fair. This does not mean that you are not allowed to use social media when off duty, however. The best way to ensure that you respect appropriate social media standards is to look at policies of other organizations that are similar to yours, to understand what is important to them. To see social media policies from organizations such as Mayo Clinic, Sutter Health, Kaiser Permanente, and others, check out the following website: http://socialmediagovernance.com.

TIP

If you do not know about your work policies, ask your manager or communications department.

Standards for Social Media Participation

What standards are considered best practices for social media use?

Currently, there are no best-practice guidelines from nursing or health care organizations. To ensure you are acting professionally, you must understand current professional standards and recommendations for social media as well as any organizational policies. While the "best way" to use social media is not yet obvious, minimum standards for acceptable behavior are becoming clear.

"Respect for ourselves guides our morals; respect for others guides our manners."

–Laurence Sterne

What are some basic standards for using social media?

There are various ways you can use social media effectively. Following is a list of recommendations of basic standards you should consider when using social media. Be aware that these standards were developed using the principles of the Health On the Net Foundation Code of Conduct (HONcode; http://www.hon.ch/HONcode/Pro/Visitor/visitor.html) and from social media policies of health care and nonprofit organizations such as the American Red Cross, found at http://socialmediagovernance.com/policies.php. These guidelines are recommendations only and are not written by a lawyer. Remember to contact your employer and professional association if you need legal advice.

* Use disclaimers—Make it clear that you are expressing your own opinions, and that they are not reflective of your employer's opinions. Information provided should support or complement traditional information channels and not replace

medical consultation from health care organizations or providers in person. Be sure to explain how you might use any information you collect.

* Be transparent—Share information about yourself, including your educational experience, so readers know you are a credible author. Ensure that your contact information, such as your e-mail address, is available so visitors can seek clarification or support regarding content. Disclose your role (membership, employee, stockholder) with organizations that you discuss online and what forms of advertisement or compensation you receive. If you create an online profile or a website for an organization or association, be sure you have permission.

* Be accurate—Posting personal opinions online is perfectly acceptable, but make sure you do proper research and check facts regarding information you post. Ensure that any links you provide work and that reference information is accurate. Take responsibility for what you post; be sure your posts do not contain false statements, copyright-protected information, or dangerous files (for example, computer viruses).

* Be considerate—Remember, anyone may be reading and following what you are posting online. Choose your words carefully! Do not post information or use language you would not be comfortable reading aloud to your family, friends, colleagues, employers, or a lawyer. Use your own judgment. Unfair public criticism of others is not smart or professional and may do you more harm than good in the end. If you truly feel strongly about an issue, raising it with the individual or through proper channels is a better approach.

* Do not reveal confidential information—As a nurse, your primary responsibility is your patients. Treating your patients requires a relationship that involves trust; respect their trust by protecting their information. Talk about what you have learned, your professional and personal views, your values, and your opinions without using specific patient information. Also, just because patients post their information online does

not mean you are allowed to share information they have given you. Know your obligations and your professional responsibilities.

* Respect copyright laws—Sharing links and content is encouraged, but you should always give credit to the original source. Respect the laws governing copyright and fair use of materials. If you are unsure, consult a fair use guide, such as Stanford's fair-use website (http://fairuse.stanford.edu).

* Tell others about your content—Send links to your content to friends and colleagues who might be interested in reading it and ask for feedback on how to improve. Also, if you are promoting an organization, be sure to let them know; that way, they can promote it or give you special instructions—for example, how to use their logo.

* Be generous—The Internet is built on the social principles of sharing and giving credit to other valuable websites. To that end, you should provide links to content you find useful so others can find it too. Properly linking helps to ensure people get credit for their work. Your visitors find valuable content, and your work becomes more credible.

> **TIP** Be transparent. People want to know who you are and that they can trust what you are saying.

* Be a good participant—Being a nurse is a privilege. Your title affords you a position of trust with the public. No matter what you are doing online, try to remember that. Social media can help you develop a professional online presence, improve collaboration among health care professionals, and provide incredible opportunities for disseminating public health information and health care insights. Make sure you use these tools for good! Dedicating your time to learning these resources is a start. Slowly increasing your participation will

provide new ways to positively affect people's perception of nurses and knowledge about their own health.

✳ Uphold your professional, organizational, and personal values—Viewers associate the content you post online with you, your organization, and your profession. Remember the values and standards that underlie these three things. If you choose to share content that does not reflect your professional or organizational values, be clear that you represent yourself and not your profession or the organization you work for.

Frequently Asked Questions

 Are there online resources to help you create a disclaimer?

The Health On the Net Foundation's website, http://www. hon.ch, has some resources. The organization also provides accreditation for health care professionals who submit their sites with links to demonstrate they are following appropriate standards. This can help you confirm that you are adhering to the guidelines and can help convince your readers that they can trust your site.

 What can and cannot be used against you by current and prospective employers?

This is one of the most difficult questions to answer. Employers have a responsibility to ensure employees follow HIPAA. Additionally, any information employers receive about your professional conduct may affect their decision to hire you or may require them to take disciplinary actions.

What's more of a gray area is whether information found about you online tarnishes your reputation and affects your desirability as an employee (Dolan, 2009). You should avoid sharing content that might damage your reputation, such as pictures of alcohol use, shop talk, criticisms of employers, or questionable posts from friends (Dolan). Although you may not think it is fair, and that it infringes on your free speech, employers have a responsibility to protect the reputation of the organization and can only interpret content as it appears.

Should nurses connect with patients on Facebook? Should faculty connect with students?

Professional relationships require some level of professional distance. Separation of professional and personal relationships helps to clarify those relationships and keep them consistent (Dolan, 2008). It is up to you to understand how you want to use your social networks and how others might use theirs. Be aware that patients or students might post information and pictures of behavior that nurses and educators would not necessarily endorse.

Turning down a request may seem difficult, but it should not be. Simply explain how you use the website and consider offering an alternative channel if they wish to keep in touch. Your work e-mail, a professional profile on LinkedIn, or a public Twitter account are alternatives that might be more appropriate and allow you to maintain professional boundaries.

Finally, be aware that relationships change over time. Some of my professors became mentors, and long after I finished their classes, I added them to my personal social networks. Be aware of how you use your social networking site and learn to distinguish how you feel comfortable connecting with people.

Should employers be allowed to have rules on how their employees use social media?

Employers should be able to set policies for how nurses spend their time on duty at work, and they need to empower employees to be effective. They also need to control how employees represent the company outside of work. Therefore, it is fair for employers to allow access only to certain websites at work, or to request that employees use personal accounts to post information online.

That being said, employers cannot limit your freedom of speech or your right to participate in online social networks, as long as your participation does not violate HIPAA or professional codes of conduct. Nurses who wish to use social media have every right to do so. But, they must make it clear that their content reflects their own opinions.

If you feel your hospital is too restrictive with its use of social media, the appropriate action is not to complain online. Instead, schedule a meeting with your supervisor or the appropriate person at your organization to discuss changes in policy or new ideas for professional uses of social media for your organization.

 What are the legal implications of inadvertently exposing client information on a site such as Facebook?

The legal ramifications can be serious for sharing patient information and should not be taken lightly. HIPAA violations can result in loss of employment, loss of professional licensing, criminal charges, and financial penalties in extreme circumstances. This is why mentioning patient information online is no casual matter. Just because members of other professions can write online about their customers does not mean health care professionals can.

If you're not sure how you should write about what you know, consider how textbooks refer to patients. Authors do not write about a real patient; instead, they use generalized information about patient populations and hypothetical examples of patients. Sharing general information about patients who rapidly deteriorate in the intensive care unit is acceptable; writing about a gentleman you treated last week for hypovolemic shock after admitting him to your unit is not.

Is it safe to communicate about nursing on a social media site?

As mentioned in this chapter, laws and regulations restrict what information can be shared about patients' health. That does not mean nurses have to be silent, however. Social media is a great way to voice your professional and personal opinions in a respectful manner. Sharing your commentary on research, such as a nursing informatics class responding to a report on the future of nursing, is a perfect example of how nurses can use social media online.

 What level of security is ensured through the use of social media?

Different social networking sites provide users different amounts of control over their data, and nurses should maximize the use of these settings. However, no social media site can perfectly guarantee security, just as credit-card companies occasionally detect breaches in security. Nurses should be aware of this and use their own professional judgment to decide what they share online. If in doubt, always ask yourself whether you would feel comfortable reading your post in front of family, friends, or coworkers.

 How can you control what pictures people can see of you online?

Each social networking site has different preferences. Take time to learn how you can adjust your settings to prevent others from identifying you in images posted online. For guidance, review the social media site's help page, or ask a friend or colleague for assistance.

Exercises

1. Find a few nursing blogs, such as http://nursing.alltop.com. Read five different entries in the blog. Look to see if they speak professionally and whether they include a disclaimer. Write down your perception of the nurse maintaining the blog.

2. Find the website of your state's nursing body and search for the social media policy. (If you do not know the organization's web address, go to http://google.com and search the name of your organization.) If you do not find any results, try visiting http://google.com, entering the name of your nursing organization, and adding "social media policy" to your search criteria.

3. Find and read your hospital's social media policy. To find it, try using the same search technique outlined in exercise 2. If you cannot locate a policy online, ask your nursing supervisor, manager, or director about it.

4. Reflect on what you found. How did the appearance and content of each nursing site make you feel about the nurse writing it? Be sure to note what you did and did not like; this will help you think about how you want to present yourself online to others. Remember, when you write online, others will perceive you not by who you are, but by how you communicate. Next, compare what you see nurses doing online with professional recommendations and your organization's expectations. Do they align? If not, why?

4

✳

Improve the Way You Access the Internet

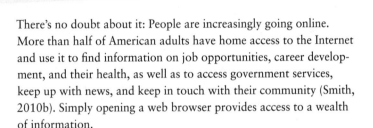

Do you:

Know there are differences among web browsers?

Start at a generic website or a customized web page?

Find more good websites than you know what to do with?

Realize there are ways to save and organize websites you find?

Use any specialized methods for search?

There's no doubt about it: People are increasingly going online. More than half of American adults have home access to the Internet and use it to find information on job opportunities, career development, and their health, as well as to access government services, keep up with news, and keep in touch with their community (Smith, 2010b). Simply opening a web browser provides access to a wealth of information.

Unfortunately, computers do not come with a guide to effective use of the Internet. Most users pick up basic skills along the way. Learning this way, however, can lead to frustration, because it does not guarantee that users will learn the important information they need to understand the Internet, nor that they will pick up tips to use it more effectively. This chapter teaches you a bit more about the Internet and provides a few tips for effectively managing all the great resources you come across.

Going Online

What ways can you access the Internet?

Web browsers are the most common way we access the Internet, but there are other ways as well. For example, there are many different applications—that is, types of software that perform a specific function—that connect to the Internet to provide a service or useful function for users. Some nurses may be familiar with applications such as Thunderbird (http://www.mozillamessaging.com/thunderbird) or Microsoft Outlook (http://office.microsoft.com/outlook), which are used to send and receive e-mail messages.

Mobile phones are another way you can access the Internet. In 2010, 82% of adults in the US owned mobile phones, and 38% of those adults have used their phone to access the Internet—up from 25% in 2009. In addition, 23% of those adults have used a social networking site, and 20% have watched a video on their mobile phone (Smith, 2010a). Mobile phone users employ apps—short for applications—to access web services while on the go.

What is a web browser?

At its most basic level, a web browser is an application that enables you to access the World Wide Web. That means that at the very least, your web browser will perform the following basic functions:

✳ Given a page's uniform resource locator (URL), more commonly known as a web address, your web browser will retrieve the information on that page (see Figure 4.1). URLs are very important because they identify one specific web page. A URL is a little like a street address. No two URLs can be exactly the same, or else the Internet simply could not work!

TIP Using an up-to-date web browser ensures that you will be able to view any type of website.

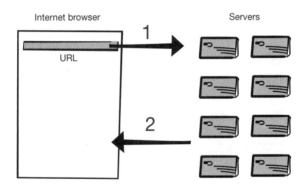

Figure 4.1: A URL gives the Internet browser the address to find a website's information.

✳ Once it accesses a web page, a web browser interprets the code on that page—that is, the language in which websites are written—and translates that code into human-readable form (see Figure 4.2). Imagine if you entered the Internet address of a page and all you could see was a bunch of letters and numbers, rather than the family photos you were expecting! Your web browser is what prevents that from happening.

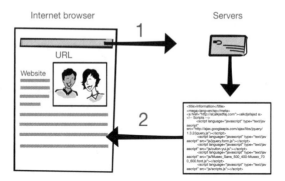

Figure 4.2: Browsers then retrieve the information and display it.

* The web browser enables you to navigate the Internet (see Figure 4.3). This can involve displaying pictures properly, activating links, and enabling you to complete forms, log in to websites, or make payments.

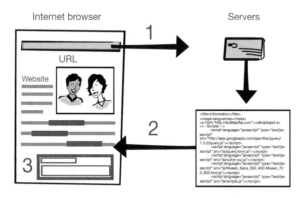

Figure 4.3: Using an up-to-date browser ensures that all elements load correctly, so you can properly view content and surf the Web.

If every web browser can do the basic functions, how are they different?

There are two important ways in which web browsers differ:

* How they perform their basic functions—How a web browser performs basic functions can improve the speed and efficiency with which you access the Internet. If you operate in a relaxed environment, you might not think using a web browser that takes 20 extra seconds to load a web page makes much difference, but those 20 extra seconds can add up over time!

* How you can modify them—Certain web browsers allow for modifications. For example, with some web browsers, you can add a plug-in, or extension—that is, an additional software component that enhances the browser's capabilities. To illustrate, Figure 4.4 shows a standard web browser; Figure 4.5 shows a browser with a plug-in installed.

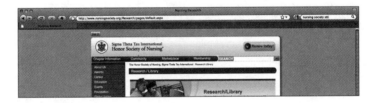

Figure 4.4: Internet browser Safari without extensions installed.

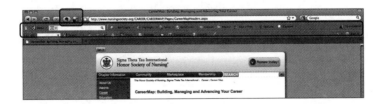

Figure 4.5: Safari with extensions for bookmarking installed.

Does it matter what web browser you use?

Even though web browsers are typically free, the browser you choose does play an integral role in how you access the Web. It's important to take a bit of time to consider what features are important to you and which web browsers offer those features.

When the Internet was in its infancy, your choice of web browser was even more important. That was because each one interpreted HTML (the language used to create web pages) in its own way. Thus, the appearance of a web page could vary drastically depending on what type of browser was used to view the page. These days, web browsers are much more standards-compliant.

"In '93 to '94, every web browser had its own flavor of HTML. So it was very difficult to know what you could put in a web page and reliably have most of your readership see."

—Tim Berners-Lee

What are the different web browser options?

A quick online search will bring up a number of web browsers. Three very popular browsers are

* Mozilla Firefox (http://mozilla.com/firefox)

* Google Chrome (http://google.com/chrome)

* Microsoft Internet Explorer (http://microsoft.com/windows/internet-explorer)

What is Mozilla Firefox?

Mozilla is a nonprofit company dedicated to protecting the accessible and secure nature of the Internet. Mozilla's Firefox, launched in 2004, is an open platform, meaning the company allows and encourages individuals around the world to contribute to the Firefox web browser's code and design. Mozilla also encourages developers to create extensions for Firefox to make the web browser more useful. Mozilla even offers rewards for people who submit information on security vulnerabilities, which is one reason Firefox was considered "unsafe" for only 9 days in 2006, compared to 284 days that Internet Explorer was considered "unsafe" that same year (Krebs, 2007). Currently, Mozilla Firefox is used for 31% of Internet traffic (StatsCounter, 2010).

Here are the pros of using Mozilla Firefox:

* Firefox is reliable and secure.

* Mozilla issues regular security updates and improvements.

* The browser is highly rated for compliance with Internet standards.

Here are the cons of using Mozilla Firefox:

* Firefox is not currently ranked as the fastest web browser.

* The browser needs to be updated regularly to ensure that new security updates work.

What is Google Chrome?

Although Google started as an Internet search company, as you will learn in this book, it now offers a lot more services than just online search. Google's business depends on users being able to use the Internet well and find what they are looking for. Using computer-engineering expertise and knowledge of web traffic and Internet standards, Google launched its own web browser, called Chrome, in 2008. Since then, Chrome has risen to handle 12% of Internet traffic (StatsCounter, 2010) and is regularly ranked as the fastest web browser (Gube, 2009).

Like Firefox, Chrome encourages development of extensions for the browser, and the number of extensions from which users can choose to improve their browsing experience has grown quickly. Chrome's only real weakness is that, being a newer web browser, it is known to be a bit more buggy—that is, subject to faults in the programming code—but regular improvements are being made.

Here are the pros of using Google Chrome:

* Google Chrome ranks as the fastest web browser and is highly compliant with Internet standards.

* A large number of extensions are available for Google Chrome.

* Rapid development means regular updates and improvements.

Here are the cons of using Google Chrome:

* Chrome is known to be a bit buggier than most web browsers.

* Using untested or conflicting plug-ins or extensions can cause problems.

* Since Chrome is new, it must be updated to fix problems.

What is Microsoft Internet Explorer (IE)?

Accounting for 48% of all Internet traffic (StatsCounter, 2010), Microsoft Internet Explorer is the most commonly used web browser—primarily because it comes pre-installed on computers running Windows software, and users do not know they can change it. IE is known among web developers as posing a challenge due to its lack of compliance with Internet standards, which means it doesn't always display features such as images, text, and embedded content properly. Because IE is a Microsoft product, development tends to take a bit longer, although a new version (IE 9) is due for release soon.

Here are the pros of using Microsoft Internet Explorer:

* Internet Explorer is a stable web browser.

* IE comes pre-installed on most Windows computers.

* Microsoft offers good customer support on the browser.

Here are the cons of using Microsoft Internet Explorer:

* Internet Explorer is not as fast as Chrome and Firefox.

* Fewer extensions are available.

* IE is updated less often, which leads to more security vulnerabilities.

Which web browser should you use?

Mozilla has started an initiative called Open to Choice. In an open letter, the CEO and chair of Mozilla wrote: "The web browser you choose is responsible for providing you with the necessary tools to manage your online life, and protect your privacy and security" (Baker & Lilly, 2010, para. 4). The key to choosing a web browser is knowing what is important to you. Here are a few points to consider:

* Security

* Speed

* Reliability

* Extensions

Nurses who are just starting out with the Internet shouldn't feel rushed to choose a web browser. Simply using the one that's already installed on your computer is fine.

If you do want to improve your browsing experience and boost security, try Firefox. This web browser is known to be stable and offers many extensions for customizing your browsing experience. Extensions will enable you to improve the way you use the Internet.

For those nurses who are feeling bold, Chrome is a great web browser. I prefer it because of its speed and the many extensions it supports. The only downside is that Chrome runs into problems now and then; when that happens, I have Firefox ready to go.

How do you find and install a new web browser?

One easy way to look at the wide variety of options and download the one you want is to visit http://www.browserchoice.eu (see Figure 4.6).

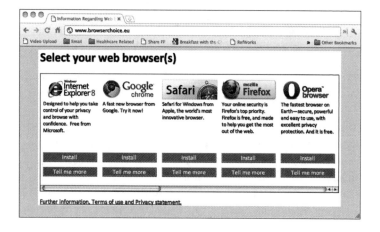

Figure 4.6: Browser Choice lets you install and learn about the differences among browsers.

Customizing Your Web Browser

How do you change the home page?

What is a home page, and how do you change it? Your web browser's home page is the first page that opens in your browser. You can change your web browser's home page by specifying which page you want to use in the browser's preferences. The options (Windows' term) or preferences (Apple's term) for each web browser will look slightly different, but they should give you some basic options for your home-page settings. To access your browser's options, click on the "Tools" menu in your toolbar, and select "Options."

What page should you choose as your home page?

There is no one-size-fits-all home page. But here are a few ideas for choosing a home page that's right for you:

* Make your home page a search engine—The Internet is an amazing source of information. Setting your home page to a search engine ensures that the first page you open will enable you to search for the information you seek.

* Resume your last web browsing session—You can set up your web browser to open the window you had open when you quit your last Internet session. That way, you can pick up where you left off.

* Choose your favorite website or news resource—This helps you stay current with news and information that is important to you.

* Create a customized website to serve as your home page— With this dashboard option—that is, one page where you can access information from a variety of sources—you can obtain information that is relevant to you from a variety of sources, right when you log on. This might include weather information, news, stock updates, and the like. You can even integrate information from your social networking sites or e-mail client.

How do you personalize your home page?

Truly creating a home page meant just for you takes a few more steps but is relatively easy. The first step is to select a personalized home page service—that is, a web service that enables you to aggregate customizable information and news. Here are a few options:

* Netvibes (http://netvibes.com)

* iGoogle (http://www.google.com/ig)

* myYahoo! (http://my.yahoo.com)

With most of these services, you set up your personalized home page using a wizard—that is, an automated process that steps you through the setup procedure. You input your interests (for example, "crafts knitting") or your professional focus (e.g., "pediatric nursing"), and the web service tries to pull in information related to those topics from a variety of sources. The result is a dashboard-style page that can help you stay up to date with the latest research and news, as well as view important information such as your local weather forecast.

As a final step, remember to change your web browser preferences to use your customized page as your browser's home page.

Organizing What You Find Online

Is there a way to keep track of websites you like?

As you explore the World Wide Web, you will no doubt find many websites that interest you. Now you need a system to help keep all those sites organized.

Fortunately, every web browser comes with the ability to bookmark websites. A bookmark is literally a placeholder—a way to store a URL so you can return to that same page again, much the way you place a bookmark in the pages of a book so you can find your place later.

Social bookmarking sites are a popular solution for both bookmarking problems. These sites enable you to do the following:

* Save your bookmarks online, making them accessible from any computer connected to the Internet.

* Organize your bookmarks by adding descriptions, tagging, and sorting.

* Send useful pages to others.

* Search for websites others have bookmarked and tagged.

How can you organize your bookmarks?

Of course, if you bookmark every web page you like in your browser, you'll eventually have so many bookmarks that you won't be able to find the one for the page you want to open (see Figure 4.7). You need a way to sort and retrieve the bookmarks you are looking for when you need them. Compounding the problem with using the web browser installed on your computer to bookmark sites is that if you switch to a different computer, you won't have access to those bookmarks.

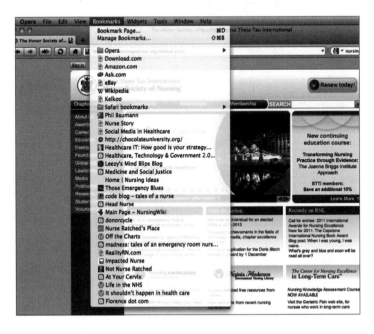

Figure 4.7: Bookmarks on your computer can easily become overwhelming to manage.

What is tagging?

In context of social bookmarking, tagging enables you to add descriptive tags to a web page. Think of tags as being like little sticky notes or labels. Tagging allows you to search your bookmarks for keywords such as "nursing," "ECG," "knitting," "cats," or "video" (see Figure 4.8). In addition, other people on social bookmarking sites such as Delicious (http://delicious.com) and Diigo (http://diigo.com) can search for tags that others have added to their public bookmarks.

TIP When you find a new site you like, save it with a bookmark. Better yet, use a social bookmarking tool to save, sort, and share it.

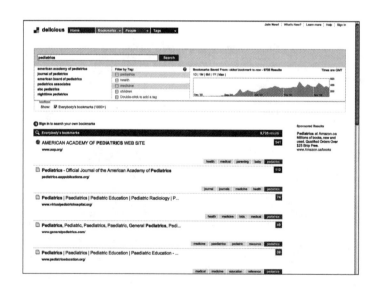

Figure 4.8: Not only does bookmarking help you keep favorite sites organized, it can also benefit others.

How does social bookmarking work?

Social bookmarking sites allow you to create a profile and use it to save bookmarks. (For help with profiles, be sure to read "Developing Your Online Profile" in Chapter 7.) There are generally two ways to bookmark a website using a social bookmarking service:

* By manually entering the site's URL and any relevant information on the social bookmarking site (see Figure 4.9).

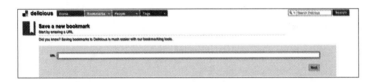

Figure 4.9: By using Delicious or other bookmarking sites, you can save URLs and add notes, tags, and descriptions of web pages.

* By installing the social bookmarking service's web browser extension, which makes bookmarking as easy as right-clicking with your mouse or clicking the new bookmarking button in your web browser (see Figures 4.10 and 4.11).

How do I install browser add-ons?

You can install extensions from the specific web services sites that created the add-on. Alternatively, many browsers have a website library of extensions for their browser that you can search through. These sites explain the add-on, and users can post ratings and comments, which will give you an idea of what to expect.

Firefox: https://addons.mozilla.org/

Chrome: https://chrome.google.com/extensions

Safari: https://extensions.apple.com/

Opera: https://addons.opera.com

Internet Explorer: http://ieaddons.com/ca/

Once you find an extension you want, click "install." You will then be prompted to confirm you want to install the add-on. This prompt may appear as "Install," "Accept," or "Allow." Once you give permission, the add-on will download and install, and you may need to restart your computer. The extension should then appear in your toolbar.

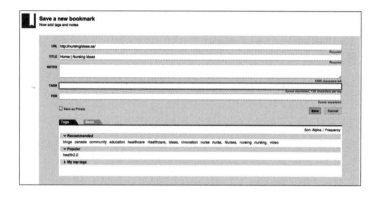

Figure 4.10: Using a browser extension for Delicious, you can right-click to bookmark the web page.

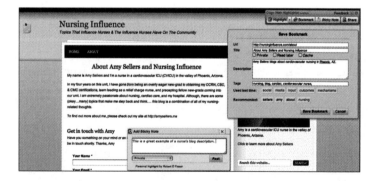

Figure 4.11: In Chrome, you can simply press a button to bookmark a page with Diigo.

How do you choose a social bookmarking tool?

Delicious was one of the first and is the largest social bookmarking tool. It focuses on offering simple bookmarking tools. Perhaps because of its age and large user base, it has developed a clean, easy-to-use interface. It also has a large public library you can search to find useful sites. Here are the benefits of using Delicious:

* It's a very stable and reliable tool.

* It's simple to use and has a large library of resources.

* It's highly used, so you can find other users with similar interests.

Diigo is the new kid on the block, if you will. A latecomer to the game, Diigo specializes in annotating the Web. In addition to the expected bookmarking capabilities, Diigo has new, helpful features— for example, tools that enable you to highlight and add sticky notes that you can view the next time you visit the site. These features are especially useful when a particular part of a long article grabs your attention, or when you have a thought you want to remember. Here are the benefits of using Diigo:

* The site's additional features are nice for remembering important information from a website.

* You can export Diigo bookmarks to Delicious, meaning you can easily use both services without duplicating work.

* You can share your annotations (highlighting and sticky notes) with other users, as well as view their annotations.

Insights & Inspiration

Teresa Heithaus, MSN, RN-BC

@NurseEducator

http://www.nsdbehindthefirewall.blogspot.com

Social media has opened a door for amazing networking opportunities with educators both within and outside of health care. In this venue, an individual can garner useful information and ideas, and learn creative uses of technology in education. Social media also offers educators the opportunity to learn about firsthand experiences and recommendations related to new web applications and software.

Becoming familiar with basic computer and social media terminology is a good place to begin. This can be accomplished by self-study or by asking an experienced colleague for advice and assistance. Both distance learning and live workshops offer certificate programs and continuing education for learning the basics of building online education programs. Some of these programs are available through nursing organizations, schools of nursing, and nurse educator entrepreneurs.

Lesson: After you learn new skills, try putting them into practice. Follow blogs of other experts, such as educators, to acquire new ideas on how to use the latest tools.

Searching

Why is searching important?

The Internet is rapidly becoming the go-to source for information. In a survey of American adults, more than 58% said they recently used the Internet at home, work, or the public library to find information (Estabrook, Witt, & Rainie, 2007). With an ever-growing source of information, individuals can't remember all the URLs. So, search engines are used to pull up websites, even ones that users frequently visit. The problem, though, is that search results are returning thousands or millions of results, which makes it harder to find the content you really want.

"The Internet is the world's largest library. It's just that all the books are on the floor."

–John Allen Paulos

What are the drawbacks of using a general search tool?

Odds are, you wouldn't go to your local Yellow Pages for information about the Revolutionary War. And, you wouldn't use a library's card catalog to find the latest Hollywood videos. Why? Because they are not the best ways to find the specific type of information you want.

General search tools must evaluate everything on the Internet, using analyses of text, links, and other features to produce a ranked list of information related to the search terms you've entered. This can make it difficult to locate the information you need.

For example, suppose you want to learn how to knit. You use a general search tool to search for the phrase "knitting tips." Now suppose that this tool uses a search algorithm that stresses the number of times a website mentions the search criteria—here, the word "knitting" and the word "tips"—together and separately. That means a yarn shop with a website that has one page with the word "tips" on it, but that lists 1,000 items whose descriptions contain the word "knitting," might well be the first result, even though the site has very little in the way of knitting tips. On the other hand, a very useful guide for beginning knitters that is posted on a person's blog might appear much further down the list. And, of course, videos and illustrations that might be very helpful in learning to knit might not appear in the top results either. This is because the search tool can't determine what type of information you really want; it simply knows what words you are looking for.

TIP Use more specific search tools to get better results in the format you prefer for your answers.

How can you improve your search for information?

One of the simplest ways users can improve their results when searching is to use some of the different tools that search engines offer. Table 4.1 compares specific search tools offered by the largest search-engine companies.

4.1 Specific types of content search using popular Internet search engines

Feature	Google	Bing	Yahoo!
General search	✔	✔	✔
News search	✔	✔	✔
Image search	✔	✔	✔
Video search	✔	✔	✔
Book search	✔		
Local search		✔	✔
Legal, research, and educational archives search	✔		
Blog search	✔	✔	✔
Map search	✔	✔	✔

Using these more specific types of search tools will change the types of results you get. Next time you are searching for an answer, consider what format you want the answer to be in.

Are there other ways to get better search results?

Absolutely. As you've learned, websites regularly include search features to help users find the information they are looking for. If you did the exercises in Chapter 2, "Understanding the Basic Building Blocks of Social Media," you will recall that you can search for information within these websites. For example,

* Social bookmarking sites—You can search these for websites that have been tagged by other users and classified according to the information they contain. A description of the website or page may also be included on the social bookmarking site.

* Video site—Searching is a great way to find videos about a certain topic. There are videos covering a wide range of topics, with some even providing instruction.

* Images—You can find images easily on specialized sites such as CompFight (http://compfight.com) or Flickr (http://flickr.com). These sites can be useful if you don't know what something looks like or if you are looking for a picture to use in a presentation or to educate a patient or colleague.

* Documents—You can find everything from PDFs to PowerPoint slides on sites such as Slide-Share (http://slideshare.net) or Scribd (http://scribd.com). You can use these documents as learning tools, for research, to see how others have presented topics in the past, or to find examples to follow.

TIP

When you find great resources, share them with people who can benefit from them.

As you begin to use more websites, you will learn their functions and their specialty areas. Remember to use your bookmarking tools to return to websites you've visited!

Exercises

1. What web browser do you use? Visit http://browserchoice.eu to learn about other Web browsers. Try installing one and comparing the experience to your current browser.

2. Take a break. Open your web browser and use the tips on searching to look for information on your interests and hobbies. The more you practice using different ways to search for information, the easier it will be when you need to find information quickly.

5

*

Dealing With the Overload

Do you:

Think you suffer from information overload?

Have a dysfunctional relationship with your e-mail?

Have more than 100 e-mails in your inbox?

Need a better system to get things done?

Know how to easily get information you need to stay up to date?

One of the largest barriers to change is limited time. Whether it is a new protocol being adopted in a nursing unit or keeping up with the latest research, it seems there is never enough time!

Learning about social media takes time, but it's important to remember that it can save time over the long run. Additionally, it can increase the impact of what you spend your time doing. That's because social media expedites the sharing of information and the rate at which information is published.

This chapter is targeted at helping you understand information overload and the importance of prioritization and time management. It also teaches you to handle the inflow of information.

Information Overload

Is more information better?

When the amount of available information increases, so does the amount of information that is relevant to you. While you might not be interested in the weather report for every city in your country, the weather information where you live is very important to you (of course, you have to be able to find it first). The same rationale should carry over to your area of nursing. Overall, the amount of knowledge and research in nursing is increasing. You may not be interested in it all, but finding the information related to your area of practice can positively affect your work and therefore patient outcomes.

Of course, not all information is useful. For example, you don't necessarily want to know when someone on Twitter is, say, hungry—unless, of course, the person who posted it was your child or some other family member. Similarly, a message about the future of nursing and leadership might interest a nurse but be of no interest to a movie maker. Fortunately, most social media services enable you to filter out content that doesn't interest you.

How did information overload start?

The idea that information overload is new is a lie we like to tell ourselves. Think about the great libraries of ancient civilizations, such as the one in Alexandria. How is that different from our local library branch, or even the Library of Congress? No one could ever hope to walk in and somehow take in all that information.

We think information overload is a new phenomenon because the speed of information growth is increasing. Internet consultant Clay

Shirky (2008) points out that information has always been increasing, and the information versus time graph has always been going up and to the right.

To support this assertion, let's look at what people had access to in 2009 (Xplane, 2009):

* 1,000,000 new books

* 1,000,000,000,000 websites

* 65,000 iPhone apps

* 10,500+ radio stations

* 5,500+ magazines

* 200+ cable TV networks

Clearly, there is no way to take in all the information that is out there. Increasing amounts of information mean we need to find ways to get the information that matters most to us. That's where filters come in.

Why has the amount of information increased?

The massive increase in information seen in recent years is due in large part to the removal of cost barriers. Costs acted as counterweights for information growth in the past. The printing press and stamps are examples of cost barriers, one for publishing and the other for sending messages. In our digital age, those costs are greatly reduced, if not eliminated entirely. This is what Shirky calls filter failure (2008). Our increased ability to publish and communicate with each other has changed who is responsible for filtering information. No longer is there one newspaper where an editor filters the stories. Now there are thousands of news sources, and we can become the editor.

How can I manage all this information successfully?

If living with an excess of information is a reality, you need to develop systems to cope with it. Here are the key parts of a successful information pipeline:

* Watch how you spend your time—Learn what web services you like to use and try to understand how and when they can be useful. Knowing when Facebook is not useful can be as important as recognizing when it can be useful. In an age where everyone can publish, there are numerous options for your time; do everything you can to spend it wisely.

* Create an inflow of information you need and want—Seek out the format (text, audio, video) of information you prefer on topics you want to learn more about or keep up to date with. Web services offer many different types of information and ways of sharing it, from presentation slide decks to microblogs, and with each format come even more topics to choose from. Everyone has interests, but that does not mean you need to keep up to date with them all. Follow people on Twitter who are in your field or you know, subscribe to podcasts that will teach you about topics you need to know, and avoid adding anything you do not need.

* Make sure to have a plan for saving and sharing information—Finding information is only half the battle; being able to find it again and sharing it with others is the other half. Social media is about developing relationships and your professional profile online. Sharing useful information with others can develop your expertise and is a great way to help others find quality resources.

Managing Your Time

You're already too busy at work. How does social media fit into your life?

As busy as they are, nurses must constantly prioritize. If your patient doesn't come first, then you (and the patient) are in serious trouble.

But eating is important too, as is filling out forms, communicating with your supervisor, remembering your sister's birthday and meeting up with an old friend. There are various reasons that we need to perform a variety of different tasks, social media included. The fact is, as a nurse, life is full of infinite demands on your finite amount of time. You need to think of social media as one of life's demands and get it sorted in your list of priorities.

How do you start prioritizing your time?

This is a problem for everyone, not just nurses. Many studies show that the human brain cannot remember everything we want it to remember. In fact, according to researchers, the human brain can only remember about seven things at once, give or take one or two. That means you can only think of a fraction of what you need to do without starting to forget items on the list. This probably explains why most nurses have pockets crammed full of notes, from vital signs to fluid in/outs. So the first step to prioritizing your time is writing down everything you need to do.

TIP If you don't prioritize what you need to get done, life will quickly get stressful!

What are the best ways to prioritize what you have to do?

Author Stephen Covey (2004) talks about how people often do things in the wrong order. That is, they tend to organize items on their to-do lists either in the order in which tasks are identified or by their due date. Covey, however, suggests that you take a different tack: Prioritize tasks on your to-do list first by importance and second by due date. This makes it easier to identify what needs to be done first. Of course, the trick then becomes to learn to move on to important tasks that are not due soon before handling not-important tasks that are due soon.

TIP Write down a list of what you need to do and prioritize it.

What does prioritization have to do with social media?

Every new form of communication and media comes with new demands on your time. Social media is no different. It would be easy to spend all day reading books in a library, without getting anything done. Similarly, you can spend hours online and not get your work done. But if you prioritize, set goals, and plan what you want to accomplish, then social media becomes a powerful tool. Pausch (2007) recommends this mental checklist when considering taking on new tasks:

TIP

A simple online search can help you find strategies for prioritizing.

* Why am I doing this? What is my goal?

* Why will I succeed?

* Am I doing the right things?

* What will happen if I don't do this?

Managing Your Inbox

Do more social media accounts mean more messages in your inbox? Yes, many social media services include messaging services to enable users to contact each other—which means if your inbox is already overflowing, it will be even fuller once you begin using social media. If this seems like a source of added stress, think about it this way: Having all those messages land in your inbox means you won't miss any of them. If you simply deal with them when you have the chance, they should empower you, not imprison you.

How can you tell if you're using your inbox effectively?

The curricula for most nursing schools don't cover how to effectively deal with e-mail, and few workplaces offer seminars on the subject. That's too bad, because using e-mail to communicate has become increasingly common, both in our personal and work lives.

The fact is, there are many ways to manage your e-mail inbox effectively. Everyone deals with e-mail a bit differently; there's no one "best way." There are, however, some signs that the way you deal with your inbox is not ideal. Here are eight indications of an out-of-control inbox:

* The number of e-mails in your inbox never goes down.

* Your only organization system is "read" or "unread."

* When you open your inbox, there is a mix-and-match pattern of open and unopened e-mails.

* When you open your inbox, you can't remember where you left off.

* Thinking about e-mails is stressful. You always feel like you've forgotten something important.

* You feel compelled to check your messages to see if there is anything urgent, but after quickly reading them, you decide you can just deal with them later.

* You use your inbox as a to-do list.

* The sound your e-mail program makes when you receive a new message interrupts you during work, so you check your inbox, but then you usually decide to deal with the e-mail message later.

Every time you open your inbox, you have new messages. How can you keep up?

When you first start using e-mail, getting a message is exciting. But that excitement soon fades as more and more messages flood your inbox. Soon, you find yourself overwhelmed. Smart phones only compound the problem; they enable you to check your e-mails on the go, but you still don't have time to do anything about them!

Continually checking your e-mail to see if there is anything you need to do, and then leaving the messages in your inbox, is not helpful. Why? First, it wastes time. You end up re-reading e-mails, and you quickly become disorganized. Second, e-mails get

TIP

Read it once, then do something with it and move on.

buried. Over time, they fade away, and nothing gets done.

When it comes to any piece of information—whether it's e-mail, regular mail, a form, a brochure, whatever—the trick is to read it once, deal with it if you need to, and then put it in its proper place by filing it, recycling it, or trashing it. If you know you won't have time to deal with the messages in your inbox, don't check it.

Are there any strategies for clearing out your inbox?

One great way to manage your inbox is called Inbox Zero. Merlin Mann (2007) developed the idea when he noticed he was constantly overwhelmed by e-mails but not getting anything done, even though he was continually checking his inbox.

What is Inbox Zero?

The idea behind Inbox Zero is you have a limited amount of time, and spending it reading e-mail is not the same thing as doing work. Simply reading your e-mail and not acting on it is like having a restaurant staff that spends all its time taking orders and not making the food. Instead, you need to decrease the amount of time you spend checking your inbox, and focus your time on work—the important things in life you need to accomplish (some of which come to you through e-mail).

A major tenet of Inbox Zero is to read each e-mail only once. Of course, this doesn't mean you can never read an e-mail again; it's just that you should make every effort to immediately deal with the e-mail. After reading an e-mail, you should take one of five actions (Mann, 2007):

* Delete it.

* Defer.

* Reply.

✳ Delegate.

✳ Do it.

How do you actually get your inbox to zero?

As difficult a task as it may be, getting your inbox to zero simply takes time and hard work. Trust me, I know: I spent a few months whittling my inbox from 3,000+ e-mails down to zero, and keeping it that way involves a daily effort.

If you follow these steps, you too can take control of your inbox and get more done:

✳ Delete it...or archive it. Quickly skim the sender and subject of the e-mail message. If the subject says "101 Ways to Nirvana" and the message is from Internet Guru.com, ask yourself: Do I have to read this e-mail? Remember, time is money and money is time. If you don't need to read it, delete it. (The fastest way to delete an e-mail message is to simply click Delete.) Alternatively, if you're worried you might need it someday, just move it to a special folder. For example, you might create a folder called "Old E-mails" for just this purpose. Or if you use a service such as Google, you can archive the e-mail; that way, you can use the Search function to find it later if need be.

✳ Defer. Sometimes, an e-mail requires you to do something that you don't have enough time or information to do right then. In that case, the task should go on your to-do list so you can handle it later. Remember, your inbox is not your to-do list; it offers no way to prioritize your tasks except by date.

✳ Respond. Some e-mails simply require you to answer a question or provide some information. For these, take the time to write that reply right away, and then delete it.

✳ Delegate. Often, people send requests for information or action to the wrong person. When reading an e-mail, consider whether you are the right person to deal with the task or request associated with that e-mail. If not, reply with as much information as possible on how to contact the correct person.

* Do it. If the task associated with an e-mail can be accomplished quickly and easily, take a few minutes to do it. Pay that bill, call and order the cake for your boss's surprise party, or whatever it is. Get it done, and get the message out of your inbox.

Creating a Knowledge Stream

What is a knowledge stream?

Once you get a handle on the incoming demands, you need to find a way to manage the growing amount of information online. With more than 1 trillion websites on the Internet, there are clearly news sources that are important to you. The trick is to make information come to you—that is, to create a knowledge stream—so you spend your time reading the relevant news rather than trying to find it.

You can create your own knowledge stream in different ways:

* E-mail newsletters

* RSS feed readers

* Podcast subscriptions

* Facebook fan pages

* Following experts and companies on Twitter

Insights & Inspiration

Carole R. Eldridge, DNP, RN, NEA-BC

@nerdnurse

www.nerdnurse.com

Nurse peers and students often ask me how I keep up with the mountains of nursing and health care research, trends, best practices, and latest evidence. For me, the key is information aggregators—those free services that pull information from a variety of sources and condense it into quickly digestible bits.

Medscape, for example, sends a daily e-mail news alert of top medical stories in my favorite specialties. The American Nurses Association e-mails daily links to information of interest to nurses. Many journal publishers offer regular e-mail digests of articles and highlights. I can customize the list of topics I want to read about, so I don't have to wade through excessive amounts of data.

These services aren't complicated or time-consuming to manage. It takes me only seconds to open the e-mail, scan through the headlines, and decide if I want to read further. If I have time, I follow the links immediately and read or save the articles to my computer. During busy weeks, I might save the reading for a spare hour on the weekend. Doing this keeps me in the know, which makes me a better nurse.

Lesson: Every nurse has a responsibility to keep up with the frequent changes in health care. An easy way to do this is to sign up for information aggregators that deliver condensed information on topics you care about to your e-mail inbox every day.

How can you use e-mail in your knowledge stream?

One of the easiest and most convenient ways to keep up with information is to sign up for e-mail news updates. You can subscribe to various types of updates, with each site providing you different options. Pay attention to websites with quality information that you find useful, and look for subscription options. You can usually find a link or icon that you can click to subscribe via e-mail (see Figure 5.1).

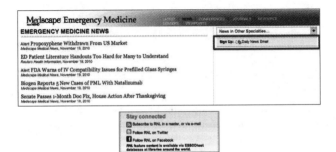

Figure 5.1: When visiting websites with useful information, look for ways that you can stay up to date.

What is the downside to using e-mail as a news source?

TIP

Don't be afraid to unsubscribe to e-mail notifications.

One of the dangers of e-mail subscriptions is that the messages can start piling up in your inbox, unread, and obscuring important e-mails that you need to deal with. Make sure to use this option judiciously. Don't be afraid to unsubscribe if you notice you are not getting much value from a news source. Just because a publisher or advertiser has your e-mail address doesn't mean it has the right to send information you don't want.

What are the alternatives to e-mail subscription?

As you use the Internet more and more, you will see that publishers are providing new ways for you to stay up to date with their information—most notably, using social networks. For example, many news sources enable you to keep up with stories using sites such as Twitter and Facebook (see Figure 5.2). When subscribing to a site, you can decide which subscription option is best for you.

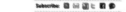

Figure 5.2: Subscribing by e-mail is just one of many ways to keep up with information.

What is an RSS feed?

In the early days of the World Wide Web, people had to visit each website they wanted to view individually, entering each URL in their web browser to check for updates. Even if you were visiting only a few websites, this became quite time-consuming. And of course, as the number of sites you wanted to view increased, so did the amount of time you wasted checking each one.

Really Simple Syndication (RSS) solves this problem by checking for updates to sites automatically and sending those updates, or feeds, to a special application called an RSS feed reader. (Google Reader is a popular example.) Users who subscribe to RSS feeds can simply open their RSS feed reader to check for new stories. The result: You spend time reading news rather than finding it. Figure 5.3 illustrates the RSS paradigm.

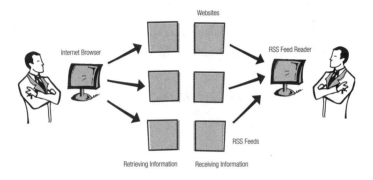

Figure 5.3: By using subscriptions, you can spend time reading information, not looking for it.

What are the advantages of using RSS feeds rather than e-mail?

Using an RSS feed reader is preferable to receiving e-mail updates because the updates on the news reader do not appear in your e-mail. Just like a newspaper or magazine, you can put aside your RSS feed reader until you have time to read it. If you get too busy on Tuesday, you can simply read the news on Wednesday; all the old news will still be there, if you really want to dig through it. Then, when you need to focus on work, you won't be distracted by news updates in your e-mail inbox.

How do you get started using RSS?

Starting to use RSS involves a three-step process:

1. Create an account.

2. Add RSS feeds.

3. Open the feed reader and read your feeds.

How do you create an RSS account?

To create an RSS account, follow these steps:

1. Direct your web browser to an RSS feed reader site. This example uses Google Reader (http://google.com/reader).

2. Click the Create an Account button.

3. Enter your information.

As shown in Figure 5.4, your account is set up, but there are no feeds yet. To learn how to add feeds, read on.

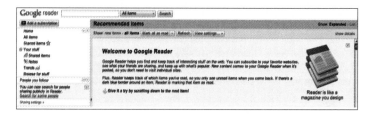

Figure 5.4: Google Reader can help you easily subscribe to and organize your RSS feeds.

How do you add RSS feeds to your feed reader?

You can add RSS feeds to your feed reader—in this example, Google Reader—in a couple of different ways:

* By searching for feeds from within the feed reader. To do so using Google Reader, click the Add a Subscription button, type your search criteria in the field that appears, and click

Add. Google Reader returns a list of feeds that matches your criteria (see Figure 5.5); click a feed's Subscribe button to subscribe to it.

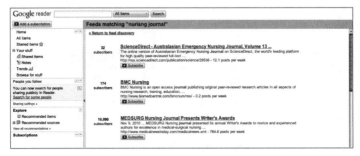

Figure 5.5: Google Reader can even help you find feeds to subscribe to.

✳ By copying the URL for a feed from its website and pasting it into your feed reader. To do so, select the feed's URL and copy it (see Figure 5.6). Then, in Google Reader, click the Add a Subscription button, paste the URL in the field that appears, and click Add (see Figure 5.7).

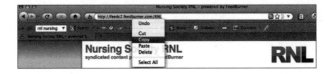

Figure 5.6: Simply copy the feed's URL to add it to your RSS feed reader.

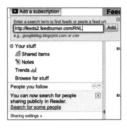

Figure 5.7: Pasting the URL into the feed reader tells it where to look for new stories.

How do you read feeds?

After you have subscribed to RSS feeds, updates to those feeds will appear in your reader. With Google Reader, you read a feed's updates by clicking the feed's name in the Subscriptions list on the left side of the screen; the updates appear on the right (see Figure 5.8).

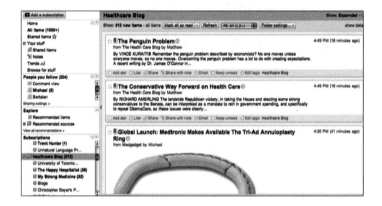

Figure 5.8: After adding subscriptions, it is easy to skim through headlines to find articles that are worth reading.

Here are a few tips for keeping up with your feeds:

You don't have to check your feeds every day. Although some people like to read their feeds daily, others prefer every other day, every few days, or weekly. See what works for you.

* Skimming is OK. You don't have to read each new entry thoroughly. You just want to be aware of what is happening and spot articles that are worth slowing down to read.

* Don't read everything. Look at the titles and only read articles that you are really interested in or that you might find useful.

* You don't have to memorize it. Click on the article to visit the website and bookmark it to come back to later if it is worth saving.

* Make it leisurely. Use this time to relax at the end of a long
day or to fill some spare time.

What else can you do with your RSS feed reader?

Google Reader is a powerful tool that can do much more than simply pull in feeds. Here are some of the features I have come to love:

* Sort. Putting RSS feeds into specific folders can help you sort
information (see Figure 5.9). For example, you might create
one folder for work-related feeds (i.e., "emergency nursing")
and one for personal interests (i.e., "knitting" or "technology
news").

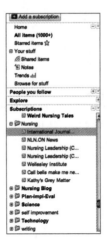

Figure 5.9: Organizing your subscriptions prevents them from getting
out of control.

* Translate. Google Reader can translate RSS feeds. If you want
to subscribe to information from a website published in another language, Google Reader can automatically translate it
(see Figure 5.10).

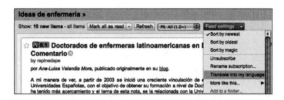

Figure 5.10: Learning a new language is no longer a requirement for keeping up with websites in other countries.

When should you use your RSS feed reader?

There are really only two times when you need to use your RSS feed reader:

1. When you need to subscribe to a new feed

2. When you need to catch up on news

Other than these two times, there is no prescription for when to use your reader. Varying when you use it, how often, and how long might be useful. It's OK to experiment until you find the right balance.

What is a podcast, and how is it useful?

RSS feeds are great for keeping up on your reading, but what if you want to subscribe to audio or video content? That's where podcasts come in. A podcast is a series of audio or video files that are released online. When you subscribe to a podcast, each episode of that podcast is downloaded automatically as it is released. You can listen to or watch the podcast using your computer or transfer it to a portable device.

Increased access to affordable technology means that podcasts aren't produced only by large organizations. That means more and more podcasts focus on increasingly niche topics.

This new form of media has a number of benefits. For one, it provides an alternative for those who prefer audio or video content over text. In addition, you can listen to podcast content on devices such as iPods and MP3 players. That means you can use time you spend in your car running errands or time you spend exercising to catch up on information that is important to you.

How do you get started using podcasts?

Manually checking all the websites that produce audio and video content you want to watch would take too much time. It's much easier to subscribe to podcasts and let your computer do all that work, automatically. One of the easiest ways to do this is by using a free application called iTunes (see Figure 5.11). In addition, you can use a number of other applications for this purpose.

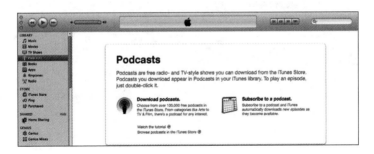

Figure 5.11: iTunes organizes your podcasts into their own section of your iTunes Library.

To download and install iTunes on your computer, point your web browser to http://apple.com/itunes/download, click the Download Now button, and follow the onscreen instructions.

How do you subscribe to a podcast?

At first, you will not have any podcasts to listen to; you will need to subscribe to some. iTunes will then download the most recent episodes for you. You can subscribe to a podcast in a couple of different ways:

 * By searching for feeds on the iTunes store. To do so, click
   the iTunes Story entry in the left pane. Then, in the Search
   field located in the upper-right corner of the screen, type your
   search criteria. iTunes displays a list of matches (see Figure
   5.12). To see more information about a podcast, click it; a list
   of episodes appears. To subscribe to a podcast, click its Subscribe Free button; iTunes downloads the most recent episode.
   Alternatively, download a specific episode by clicking its Free
   button.

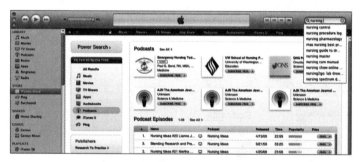

Figure 5.12: The menu on the left tells you what information you looking at, in this case the iTunes Store. The Search field is in the upper right-hand corner.

 * By copying the URL for a feed from its website and pasting it
   into iTunes. To do so, select the feed's URL and copy it. Then,
   in iTunes, open the Advanced menu and choose Subscribe to
   Podcast (see Figure 5.13). Paste the URL into the iTunes dialog box (see Figure 5.14).

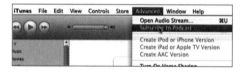

Figure 5.13: Select Subscribe to Podcast to manually enter a podcast feed.

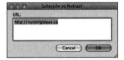

Figure 5.14: Paste the feed address into the dialog box and press OK to begin your subscription to a new podcast.

How do you listen to or watch a podcast?

To view podcasts that iTunes has downloaded, click the Podcasts entry on the left side of the screen. A list of podcasts to which you have subscribed appears under the Podcasts entry; click the podcast you want to watch or listen to. iTunes displays episodes of that podcast in the pane on the right, marking unwatched episodes with a blue dot (see Figure 5.15). To watch or listen to an episode, click it, and then click the Play button in the upper-left corner of the screen.

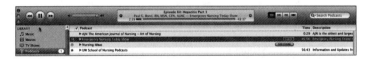

Figure 5.15: When you subscribe to a podcast, iTunes will download the latest episodes and put them in the podcast section of your iTunes Library.

How do you transfer a podcast to a listening device?

If you have an iPod, iPad, or iPhone, you can copy your podcast to it. Alternatively, you can set it to automatically sync with iTunes—transferring new podcasts to your device and removing podcasts you have already watched or listened to. Here's how:

1. Attach your iPod, iPad, or iPhone to your computer using the appropriate cable.

2. In iTunes, click the entry on the left for your iPod, iPad, or iPhone.

3. The right side of the screen changes to include information about your device. Click the Podcasts link along the top of the screen (see Figure 5.16).

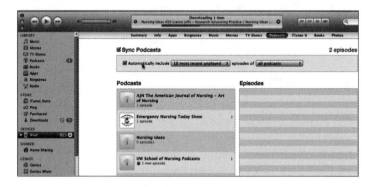

Figure 5.16: iTunes can be configured to automatically sync podcasts, to update your shows anytime you connect your device.

1. Set your sync options.

2. Click Sync. iTunes syncs your device.

When should you listen to podcasts?

Once you find a few podcasts you like, experiment with how you like to listen to them. Are you really trying to learn something from them, or do you just want to keep up with news? This will determine how much you need to focus on what you are listening to. Here are some ideas for when you could listen to a podcast:

* While using a treadmill

* During car trips

* When out shopping

* When commuting to or from work

* At the gym

There is no right way to listen to a podcast; they are just another way to consume information that is important to you. Whether you listen to university lectures or comedy acts, just be sure you enjoy them and get something out of them.

Frequently Asked Questions

 What should you do if everyone expects you to always check your e-mail?

In the past, unless it was an emergency, people would not call you at 9 p.m. on a Sunday. It just was not done. The challenge with e-mail, especially in work or professional relationships, is that people can contact you whenever they want. If you are in a professional situation where you're expected to always be available, you may need to talk to your supervisor about his or her expectations. If you really want to be bold, use that conversation to explain how checking e-mail might make you less productive, because doing so prevents you from focusing on your work.

 What does social media do for you, other than give you more things to do?

Social media gives you more tools. Whether for relationship building or collaborating on a project, these tools can save you time. As counterintuitive as it may be, more can mean less—less time wasted. Using these tools, you can spend more time working on your goal and stay up to date with family, best practices, or both, depending on how you choose to use them.

 What are e-mail filters?

E-mail clients such as Gmail allow you to create rules for in-coming messages. For example, any message from the e-mail address @facebook.com could automatically be sent to a folder called "Facebook" and never appear in your inbox. This enables you to sort your e-mails before you see them. Then, when you have time, you can check these folders for information of interest to you. This can be especially useful for e-mails from social networking sites. These sites often send you notifications to encourage you to go to their website, which can steal even more of your time.

You have too many e-mails to ever achieve Inbox Zero. What do you do?

If you have a hopelessly huge pile that you're simply not going to be able to get through, you may have lost the battle. However, that does not mean you cannot win the war. Why not take all your e-mails and put them in a new folder called "Old Inbox"? Ta-da! You now have an empty inbox! Now, anytime you check your e-mail, deal with it immediately. Then spend your extra time working through some of your old e-mails. If you're worried you might miss something important, don't be; odds are that was going to happen with your old system anyway. If you really must, simply explain the situation to your colleagues and family and ask them if there is something they need from you. Then just stick with your new system.

What is the best system for sorting your e-mails?

There is no perfect taxonomy or categorization system that will help you to perfectly sort e-mails into the "correct folder." Just remember the advice to keep it simple. A good strategy might be to have two folders—one called "Work" and one called "Personal." Then you might create new folders for any projects or committees of which you are a part. This will help you to quickly sort e-mails. It also makes it easy to review information before events, meetings, or teleconferences.

What RSS feeds do you recommend?

My selection of RSS feeds is a little biased toward technology sites. The key is to find sites that put out quality content you are interested in and want to keep up with. Professional associations and nursing journals are good places to start. Another way to find good nursing content is to look at what others are reading. Bloggers regularly post links to their favorite sites, which may be of interest to readers. Check to see who or what they are reading; chances are you will have similar tastes.

Where can you find nursing podcasts?

If you have downloaded and installed iTunes, you can easily find nursing podcasts in the iTunes Store. In addition, you can search online podcast directories such as Podcast Pickle (http://www.podcastpickle.com) and Podcast Alley (http://www.podcastalley.com). Or, you can use Google to search for keywords such as "ICU" and "emergency" along with "podcast." Medic Cast (http://mediccast.com) is another great place to start. There you'll find a number of podcasts for medical professionals, including nurses.

Exercises

1. While the information in this chapter soaks in, visit YouTube (http://youtube.com) and search for "Did You Know 4.0" by xplanevisualthinking, and take 5 minutes to watch it.

2. Think about what information is important to you. What websites do you regularly visit for new information? What information source would help you stay up to date with nursing issues relevant to you and your practice setting?

3. Create an account with an RSS feed reader. Then visit your favorite websites and see if they offer RSS feeds. If they do, add them to your reader account. In a few days, visit your feed reader and see if any articles interest you.

4. Finally, it's time to deal with that inbox. Set aside 25 minutes and really focus. Don't get distracted. Use the five actions outlined by Inbox Zero to move those messages out of your inbox, and feel your e-mail anxiety fade away:

   * Delete/archive

   * Delegate

* Respond
* Defer
* Do

6

*

Developing Your Online Reputation

Do you:

Have a website?

Know when to use your personal e-mail rather than your work e-mail?

Fill in all the information you need to?

Think about how others will perceive your online posts?

Showering and putting on clean clothes before heading out to work or for a job interview seem like common sense. After all, everyone knows that how we dress and smell can affect how others perceive us. Similarly, we shift the way we speak depending on whom we are addressing. Every day, we make decisions that color how others perceive us.

When it comes to social media, others can see every piece of content you post. That means it's important to consider how your posts will affect what others think of you. This chapter talks about everything from signing up to commenting on others' posts, to make sure you represent yourself online in the best possible way and know how to develop your professional profile.

"A brand for a company is like a reputation for a person."

–Jeff Bezos

Reputation

How can the use of social media affect your reputation?

Social media spreads information, enables people to communicate, and facilitates collaboration. When you use web services, other people can read, listen to, and watch content you produce, as well as read about you in your profiles. These services also make it easier for others to see how you communicate and to directly communicate or collaborate with you. Your actions online tell other people about you, so it is important to make sure you are building your reputation in a good way.

Why does your online reputation matter?

What happens online can affect your reputation offline, both positively and negatively. Developing a positive reputation online can represent a real opportunity offline; it enables you to reap what you sow. No one, to my knowledge, has ever been fired for developing an online presence as an expert in his or her field or as an intelligent and hard-working individual. Of course, avoiding the pitfalls that result in a negative online reputation is just as important, because your career and professional reputation may be on the line.

Some people might think that you can't foster a reputation online. After all, when you're online, you can't really do anything; it is just talk. But if you've ever received a rude e-mail or been frustrated by an unhelpful reply, you can attest to the fact that these experiences affect your attitude and perception of the person on the other end of the exchange. In the same way, if someone goes above and beyond to answer your question, provide you with useful information, or share resources or contacts, you will have a completely different perception of that person. Remember, any time you click Send, Post, or Upload, the content you share reflects on you. And while reflections might not be perfect representations, they are what others see.

Having a good reputation online can be beneficial in several ways:

* You can become known for specific skills or abilities.

* You can foster interest among potential employers.

* You can help secure opportunities to fulfill career goals.

* You can force yourself to continually improve.

* People may come to you for advice or help.

* Others will understand what you do and why it is important.

* Being self-aware causes you to improve the way you communicate.

What is involved in building a positive reputation online?

Building a positive reputation online is similar to building one offline. It's complicated, and it's a combination of many little things. Unfortunately, there are not six easy steps or a magic pill. You earn a reputation, whether online or offline, over time. It consists of what you say and, more importantly, what you do. Your reputation is built on others' experiences and interactions with you.

Alvarez del Blanco (2010) notes six areas for building a positive reputation, and some basic do's and don'ts for each one (see Table 6.1).

6.1   Key characteristics for building your reputation

Characteristic	Do	Don't
Competence	Do share your expertise, knowledge, and specialized skills.	Don't be afraid to talk about what you know. Don't pretend to know what you are not sure of.
Courtesy	Do be friendly and respectful with all your communications. Do always be on your best behavior.	Don't think that if it's just one e-mail, comment, or post, it doesn't matter. Every online post represents a piece of your reputation, so it is important to make all posts positive and reflective of the image you want to project. Don't post or write a response in the heat of the moment.
Credibility	Do back up opinions with valid arguments. Do use credible sources when possible.	Don't cite "facts" that you cannot back up. Don't over-generalize or draw unfounded conclusions.
Confidence	Do feel comfortable commenting and joining online conversations where your opinions are relevant.	Don't sell yourself short and think no one wants to hear from you. Don't be overconfident and fail to listen to others.

Characteristic	Do	Don't
Responsibility	Do take accountability for what you post and for promises you make.	Don't blame others.
		Don't ignore commitments you have made.
	Do respond to people who contact you or ask you questions.	
Communication	Do continually improve the way you communicate, no matter what format.	Don't share information that might be misinterpreted.
		Don't make it the responsibility of others to understand what you are saying if you are unclear.

What web services do you need to use to build your reputation?

Even though Alvarez del Blanco (2010) lists some ingredients for building a solid reputation, there is no perfect recipe to follow. As your knowledge of current—and future—web services and tools grows, you will better understand what they can do and how they may be useful for building your reputation.

As a first step, signing up and completing a profile for any online service you want to use—LinkedIn, YouTube, Facebook, SlideShare, etc.—will help you develop a consistent online presence. People will learn more about you, which will build your reputation. You'll learn more about profiles in the next section.

"Sometimes I feel limited by people's perceptions of what I can and cannot do."

–Mira Sorvino

Profiles

What is a profile?

Nearly every web service will require you to create a user profile before you can use the service. Indeed, profiles are a core part of all social media tools. Not only does this enable these web services to learn a bit about you, it allows other users to see, evaluate, and connect with you.

TIP
Make sure any information you or your organization posts about you is accurate.

An easy way to think of a profile is simply as an advanced version of an entry in a phonebook, a photo in a high-school yearbook, or a résumé. Your profile functions as a source for relevant information about you. Someone viewing your profile can find out how to contact you or learn more about you. The best part is that you can update your profile when you change your phone number, find a new hobby, or gain new work experiences.

At first, profiles may seem complex. Complicating matters is the fact that each one is different. But as you gain more experience, it becomes easier to complete and update them. Plus, although each web service may have a different setup, the basics are the same; most profiles require a user name and varying amounts of personal or professional information.

Shouldn't your organization take care of posting your contact details online?

Employers are most concerned with their business. Even though most organizations now have a website, it may or may not have an employee directory or profiles of staff. But even if they do, you need to remember that your organization is only interested in posting information that it believes its clients will need. Most hospitals don't use their websites to help support their employees' career advancement, professional image, or other activities in which members of their nursing staff engage. It's up to you to consider how you can build your reputation and career success using the various online tools available to you.

Why do you need to fill out online profiles?

Social networking may not be the focus of all web services; however, many—especially when users publish or can comment on content—have some profile features. Content-sharing sites such as YouTube or SlideShare are great examples of this. Users may simply be watching a video, but having a profile allows them to learn more about who made a video, which is important for building credibility and reputation. Similarly, authors can evaluate and put comments received into perspective if they can identify the source of agreement or criticism.

Profiles give permission for others to find out more about you. Viewing this information will shape a person's perspective of the characteristics that build your reputation, for better or worse. By completing and improving your online profiles, you take part in shaping the impression that others have of you. You can work on improving how others perceive you—what you are capable of doing and your areas of knowledge, experience, or skills.

What are the different parts of an online profile?

At first glance, user profiles for one social media site may appear to be very different from user profiles on another site. But when you take a closer look, you begin to recognize similarities.

The truth is, most profiles share a basic anatomy. That is, the components of profiles from different social media sites accomplish similar things. It's similar to comparing the legs of humans and cheetahs. Cheetahs' legs enable them to run faster, while humans' legs allow them to stand taller. But, they serve the same general purpose—to stand, walk, and run. Table 6.2 explains what each of these components does; Figure 6.1 shows a sample profile.

(6.2) Building blocks of an online profile

Component	Purpose	Utility
Name	Shows the user's preferred name	Identifies whose profile you are viewing Indicates how that person prefers to be addressed
User name	Serves as a unique identifier for the person	Identifies a specific person on the web service May be used to direct messages to that person May be used to identify user's content or comments elsewhere on the site or on a different site
Contact info	Displays options for contacting an individual May include traditional contact information (phone, address, e-mail, etc.), and could provide clickable options such as "Contact User" or "Send Message"	Provides useful information for contacting the individual Increases the user's credibility and responsibility for the content, because his contact information is visible
Short bio	Includes a brief outline of the user's personal information or his or her reasons for using the web service	Quickly identifies important information that the user discloses about himself or herself May explain why the user is using a web service

Component	Purpose	Utility
Detailed information	Provides more detailed information about the user	Shares more about the user's personal or professional interests and experiences
		Enables others to better understand the user
Posted content	Links the profile to the purpose of the web service (for social networking sites, posted content might be status updates; for content-sharing sites, it might be videos or presentations the user has uploaded)	Enables others to easily see all the user's activities (or his or her most recent activity) on the site
		Enables others to find additional content the user has posted
		Displays a cumulative list of content shared through the web service
Liked content	Shows content this user has found interesting, noteworthy, or worth sharing (various web services may name this function differently)	Identifies the user's tastes and shares resources that he or she has found useful
		Allows users to curate content for a niche audience
		Enables others to find shared interests and exchange resources
Connections	Shows who the user is connected with on that web service	Enables users to locate people who may share professional or personal interests
		Enables users to explore mutual connections or find other shared interests and associations

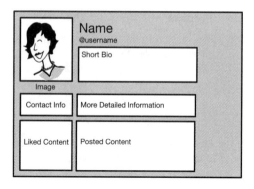

Figure 6.1: When you recognize the different components of an online profile, you see the similarities among various networking sites and web services.

Do you have to memorize all the profile parts?

While you don't need to worry about creating flash cards for the various parts of a profile—after all, it's unlikely you'll be given a pop quiz about them—it's a good idea to understand what the different components can do. This will enable you to quickly complete your profile any time you join a new social media site. You'll also learn more about what information others are looking for. Finally, knowing where to look on others' profiles will help you find the information more efficiently. Fortunately, as you use social media over time, you'll naturally become more familiar with the various parts of a user profile.

> **TIP**
> **Learn to recognize the purpose of these profile components, and think about how others will read content.**

What is the best way to fill out your profile?

Although no official research has studied how to create an optimal profile, here are a few recommendations:

* Choose a strong user name

* Use your personal, rather than your work, e-mail address.

* Be as complete as possible.

* Include a photo or other image.

* Use proper spelling and grammar.

* Consider connecting profiles from different sites.

* Understand the site's culture.

You don't have to follow these recommendations to a T, but they should act as guiding principles when you set up your profiles.

Learning how to quickly and effectively set up a profile that you feel good about and represents you well is important. Some people may argue that what you do with social media tools is more important than your profile. But, like the title page and reference section of an essay, a profile gives context and credibility to what you do with social media.

How do you choose a strong user name?

When it comes to profiles, there are two types of names:

* Your actual name

* Your user name

For your actual name, it's best to use your common first name and last name. If people know you by your maiden name or a hyphenated version, make sure to use that. Also, keep your name consistent across all social media sites. That's helpful when users try to find you on different web services. Consistency is especially important with common names—such as mine, Robert Fraser—because there are many possible nicknames (Rob, Robbie, Bob, Bobby, Bert, Bertie, etc.). The only time you might want to use different names is to differentiate between personal and professional social networking sites. For example, if your friends call you Dot, but you go by Dorothy at work, you might use Dot on Facebook and Dorothy when signing up for LinkedIn.

User names are a little different. Because web services need to be able to identify each person on the site, they require you to choose a unique user name. Here are a few do's and don'ts for choosing a user name:

* Do use your real name—If your real name is available (that is, if other people who share your name haven't beaten you to it), choosing it as your user name can help identify you to others. It will also help connect your online presence with your name when people search for you.

* Do use initials—Especially if your name is more common, including your middle initial can help you create a unique user name out of your real name.

* Do include your interests or profession—Including a reference to your passions, interests, or profession helps others identify with you and can help build relationships. For example, a user name such as caffeinatednurse is great for a blog, Twitter, or other social networking sites.

* Do be creative—If you really cannot find a name you are happy with, don't settle. Come up with something meaningful or funny. It will help you stand out and be remembered.

* Do think about how others will read it—Remember, your user name should be easy for others to remember. You want them to have a positive reaction when they read it.

* Do avoid using numbers—They aren't very memorable and don't give others useful information about you.

* Don't imitate others—Sure, you may love celebrities. But using names of other people or characters won't help you establish a unique online identity.

* Don't be unprofessional—Although you might think cutenurse is a fun username, it's not the image you want to project. Your user name reveals a lot about your identity and judgment!

* Don't be profane or offensive—Remember, this is how other people will find and address you. Don't use words that will offend others or make them uncomfortable.

If you are not sure what names are available, go to CheckUser-Names (http://checkusernames.com), where you can check more than 300 social media sites for the availability of a username. This will ensure that the one you choose is available on various sites, which is important for consistency.

Why is it important to use your personal e-mail address?

An e-mail address is the 21st-century version of letterhead. It identifies you. When you send an e-mail, your address tells the receiver who you, the sender, are; whether you are using your work or personal account; and (if you are using your work account) the organization or entity with which you are affiliated.

When signing up for social media accounts, it's better to use your personal e-mail address than your work e-mail address. There are two reasons:

* Using your work e-mail has a few risks—For one, it may be against company policy. For another, you might receive e-mail notifications about personal matters during work, which can be very distracting. Remember, your employer gave you an e-mail account for a specific reason, and there may be serious consequences if you use it in a manner that violates workplace policy. Additionally, if you leave your job, you will no longer receive account-related notifications and may lose access to the account altogether.

* Better management of notifications—Social media accounts often send e-mails with notifications and updates related to your account. Using a personal e-mail account gives you the choice of when to look at these messages. You can also open a free e-mail account for use with social media sites; that way, important e-mails won't get buried by notifications sent to your personal account.

Why is it important to complete your profile?

An incomplete profile can be worse than no profile at all. Why? Because when others visit your profile, they are looking for information about you. If they don't find what they need, they can feel frustrated.

Whenever you open an account, be sure to take at least 10 minutes to fill out as much information as you can (and feel comfortable providing). If 10 minutes is not enough to complete the entire profile, take as much time as you need to wrap it up or, if you can't spare another minute, remember to finish the remaining pieces later.

Some social media sites help you remember to complete your profile (see Figure 6.2). Others even provide basic coaching to help you populate your profile.

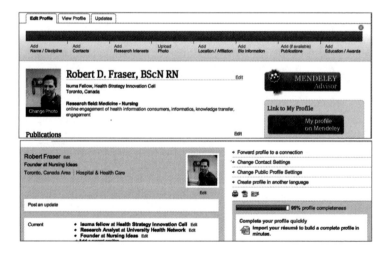

Figure 6.2: Web services encourage you to complete your profile. For example, LinkedIn (top) and Mendeley (bottom) tell you what percentage of your profile is complete.

Why is it important to include a photo or other image?

One of the most common features of profiles is the option to include a picture. Unfortunately, many people do not bother to add one (except on social networking sites). Being able to identify a profile by name is helpful, but a picture can be even more meaningful. It helps to truly connect you to your profile.

You should have one digital photograph that you can use as your default picture for new profiles. Having it handy—somewhere on your computer where you can find it easily—can help you check this step off in your first 10 minutes of setting up your profile.

If you do not have an image you like, you have a couple of options. One is to ask someone you know to take a picture you can use. Make sure you are the only person in the picture and that it is a close-up; having multiple people in the picture can be confusing and make it harder for others to easily identify you. Alternatively, you can create an avatar—a representation of yourself, as shown in Figure 6.3—that you can use in profiles. This is one way to avoid uploading an image of yourself while still helping others to easily recognize your profiles. One site that enables you to create custom avatars free of charge is Face Your Manga (http://faceyourmanga. com).

Figure 6.3: An example of an avatar.

Are spelling and grammar important?

To create a social media profile, you don't have to be able to write sonnets or prose. Spelling and grammar are important, however. When you are building your online reputation, the quality of your work speaks for itself, and one of the natural measures is your ability to communicate. Everyone is human, and a typo or two is easy to make—but it's just as easily fixed when you notice it. More important is basic proofreading of what you post to make sure it can reasonably be understood. This principle is even more important when you are specifically using social media tools to build your professional reputation. When posting information on LinkedIn or videos on YouTube, make sure you double-check them to make sure you do not detract from your hard work with a simple-to-fix typing error.

Should you connect profiles from different sites?

Many social media services include an option for you to add your website address with your other contact information. Even if you don't have your own website or maintain your own blog, you might still have a website you can add. After all, each profile you create on a social media site is your website, in a manner of speaking. You control what is posted there and what perspective it might give people. If, for example, you have completed a LinkedIn profile, you can copy the URL for that public profile and paste it in the website field when entering your contact information for other social media sites. That way, if people want to see more information about you, they can explore the site you provide.

When filling out your profile for other social media sites, you may also be asked to enter information about your Twitter, Facebook, and LinkedIn accounts, so that content from those sites can be posted on the new social media site. In this situation, it's best to consider the fit between the two sites. Do they have similar purposes? If not, don't feel pressured to include the information. For example, if LinkedIn allows you to submit YouTube details so that videos you post on YouTube will also automatically appear on LinkedIn, you need to think about compatibility. If you are posting videos containing interviews with clinical experts who have advice for other nurses or job interview tips for students, it might be a great fit. On the other hand, if you're posting videos of your beautiful niece playing with bubbles, then probably not.

Insights & Inspiration

Lorry Schoenly, PhD, RN

@lorryschoenly

http://linkedin.com/in/lorryschoenly

I work in the invisible world of correctional nursing. Many nurses, including me at one time, do not know about the specialty practice of delivering nursing care in jails and prisons.

When I discovered social media several years ago, I could see that this was an excellent way to communicate to a broader audience the special issues of delivering care to the incarcerated. I provide in-depth information on my blog (CorrectionalNurse.Net) and use Facebook, Twitter, and LinkedIn groups to share news items, resources, and concerns in the field. Social media is helping me meet my goal of making correctional nursing visible to the nursing community and beyond by having a presence in a wide variety of channels.

Lesson: Start with one social media channel, and then add others as you get more comfortable. To update multiple profiles at once, you can use time-saving applications such as Ping.fm (http://ping. fm). With Ping.fm, I can use Twitter as my communication base and send tweets to Facebook and LinkedIn as appropriate. I also schedule posts through SocialOomph, so I can cover all the time zones without being continually active.

Why do you need to understand the site's culture?

Social media experts often say that using social networking sites is like being at a cocktail party. While being polite and respectful is necessary, speaking the right language can be just as important. Just as being at a cocktail party for members of a college fraternity is a lot different from attending a cocktail party with your grand-mother's country-club set, there are big differences among various social media sites. When joining a professional networking site such as LinkedIn, think business formal. In contrast, Facebook is much more business casual, if not dressed for the weekend. Look around to see how others are using the site and follow their lead until you are comfortable deciding when and how you want to stand out.

What can you do to build your reputation after you complete your profile?

After you fill out your profile, the best thing to do is to join in the conversation. Remember the cocktail party metaphor. However, creating your profile doesn't mean you have to jump right in and lead online discussions. Take a look around the website you signed up for. Find content that is interesting to you. Then start to join in the conversations.

One easy way to begin participating in conversations online, and thereby build your reputation, is to post comments on articles you read. Many sites ask for your name and e-mail address when you leave a comment; others also enable you to post a link to your website (see Figure 6.4). In this case, you can post a link to your profile. Doing this allows the author of the article or other content to find out more about you. More importantly, when you comment on an article and include a link to your profile, other nurses reading the article can

* See that another nurse (you) is reading the article.

* Gain an understanding of another perspective on the article from your comments.

* Find out more about you by clicking on your link and viewing your profile.

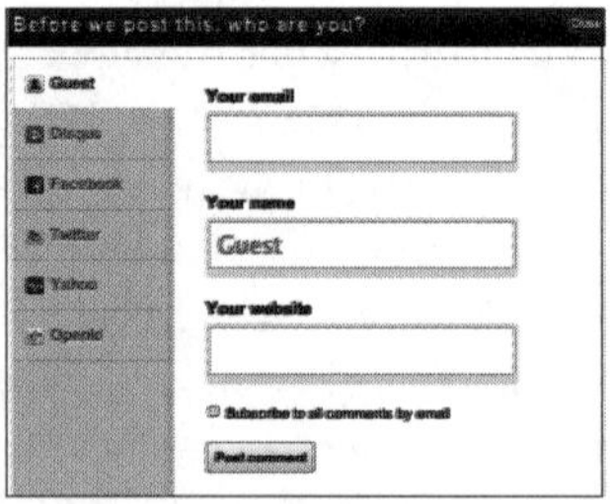

Figure 6.4: Some comment sections allow you to log in to other social services.

Another way to promote your social media profile is to include a link to it in your e-mail signature. This allows others to learn more about you through the profile. The link can also help others to see you are part of the same network and can connect there.

Frequently Asked Questions

 You don't know anyone using these social networking sites. What should you do?

Consider telling your friends or colleagues about the sites. You don't have to tell everyone; just start with people you think might benefit from using the service. If you can teach others the benefits of using the service, you will see your number of contacts on the service grow.

The other option is to go online. Facebook and LinkedIn have different features for groups and associations. Try searching online for topics or organizations that you like. You can join the groups and begin engaging in conversations online to meet other people.

 Does having an online profile really make a difference?

Using social media sometimes feels like signing up for a gym membership. Signing up and completing a profile do not create results; it takes time and effort. This does not have to be several hours a day—even small doses over time can have a large impact. Using social media can create new opportunities for you, ranging from a growing number of connections or subscribers to job or collaboration opportunities.

 Do you have to provide every piece of information a profile asks for?

No. Do not feel pressured to disclose information you are not comfortable sharing with others. Provide information only if you truly trust the web tool and think you will experience a real benefit. Information such as your home address, banking information, or information you want to keep private is yours to protect.

Transparency on the Web means being honest about your motives for participating and allowing others to gain an understanding of who you are. It does not mean you have to share every aspect of your life. Your social media profile is similar to a résumé. Some information is important to share—work experience, education, etc.—and other information is important to leave off to protect your privacy.

Will LinkedIn help you get a job?

Social media tools do not do the work for you. Having a résumé does not get you a job; what that résumé represents—your education and work experience—get you the job. Participating in social media sites such as LinkedIn can help you do things that will help you get a job. Networking with other professionals, learning about current trends and patterns in health care, and finding out about opportunities to get involved or contribute are all possible ways to use sites such as LinkedIn.

How do you stop too many people from contacting you?

Naturally, signing up for social media sites will enable others to contact you more readily. That's the whole point. It seems the real question here is how to limit your social network to a certain group with which you wish to communicate. For social networking sites such as Facebook or LinkedIn, be clear in how you want to use them; then simply explain your "usage policy" to people who contact you. Pretending someone is not talking to you or requesting to connect is rude. Simply and politely explain how you are using the tools and provide a better solution for them. For example, you might use Facebook to stay connected only with family and friends, and send others toward your LinkedIn profile to connect there.

Exercises

1. Let's take our first steps toward setting up a professional profile online. To begin, have the following handy:

   * Your résumé—This will enable you to easily fill in details from your employment background.

   * A profile picture—This should be an image that you feel comfortable using. Save it where you can easily locate it to upload later.

   * A personal e-mail account—Decide whether you want to create a separate e-mail account for receiving personal notification e-mails.

2. Pick a social media site you want to use, and create an account. To begin, open the website in your browser. If you can't decide which social media site to start with, opt for LinkedIn (http://www.linkedin.com). Then click the option for joining. It may be a Join Now button, a Sign Up link, or something similar.

3. Follow the instructions for creating the account. This may require you to provide your name, a user name, and an e-mail address. (These websites do this to make sure you are a real person.) When prompted for a user name, visit http://check-usernames.com to test the availability of user names you are considering. When you're finished, most sites will send you a confirmation e-mail; open the e-mail and click the link it contains to finalize the account.

4. Now that you have an account, it's time to populate your profile. To start, log in to your account, find the option to edit your profile, and spend some time filling in the different fields. After 10 minutes, see what your profile looks like; then decide if you want to keep adding information now or wait until later. If you put it off, don't forget to return to the site to fill out the rest of the information later.

7

*

Begin to Share Your Knowledge

Do you:

Realize you have valuable insights, knowledge, and perspective to share?

Contribute to the advancement of the professional image of nurses?

Continually develop new knowledge and keep current with best practice?

Have experience or advice that would be useful for other nurses?

Work in an area of nursing that needs to engage the public or broader profession of nursing more?

Creating a social media profile enables you to highlight who you are today. Actually participating in social media is where you can begin to have a positive impact on your community, nursing and otherwise. Sharing content through social media pushes you to engage in lifelong learning and self-reflection. Writing a blog post or preparing a video prompts you to reflect on your experience and knowledge, a process that can lead to personal growth. Producing new content can and should involve learning new and relevant information to share—in effect, forcing your to learn.

Many nurses already engage in continual learning practices and self-reflection (Mann, Gordon, & MacLeod, 2009). The benefit of using social media in the process is that your actions can ripple out, influencing others in addition to yourself. What this really means is your actions can be amplified, benefiting you in personal growth, bolstering your reputation, helping others to learn, and fostering a professional and collaborative culture in nursing. Achieving this starts when you begin to share your knowledge online. This chapter covers getting started, targeting your audience, finding your voice, and exploring a few potential mediums for sharing your content.

"Be yourself. Above all, let who you are, what you are, what you believe, shine through every sentence you write."

–John Jakes

Shifting From Attendee to Participant

What comes after signing up for online networks?

Creating a profile is a significant first step—but remember, it's only the first of many. Creating a social media profile merely enables you to be present. The next step is to participate in the exchange of ideas with others who are also online. By participating, you harness the power of Web 2.0 and allow more information to be created and shared.

What is the benefit of creating social media content?

Taking time to share your knowledge and experience is important—for you, for the nursing profession in general, and for the public. Even though we all know nurses are smart and well-educated, only 7% of the public agrees, and only 8% of that public thinks of nurses as professionals (Sullivan-Marx, McGivern, Fairman, & Greensberg, 2010).

Even though only a select group of nurses actively publishes research articles, the general value of publishing information is understood. Oermann and Hays (2002) note that writing for traditional publications enables nurses to do the following:

* Share ideas and expertise.

* Disseminate evidence and research findings.

* Create career opportunities (promotion, tenure, etc.).

* Develop personal knowledge and skills.

* Create a sense of accomplishment and personal satisfaction.

These types of benefits can also be experienced in real ways using social media. Social media, however, includes completely new tools that allow for different types of publication, sharing, and discussion among nurses. Some of the additional benefits of sharing your expertise through social media include the following:

* You can increase the speed of knowledge dissemination.

* You can increase the impact of your work by sharing it.

* You can provide new perspectives on issues related to nursing and health care.

* You can foster a dialogue before issues enter traditional publication streams.

* You can collect input from people who view or use content.

* You can improve the public's perception of nurses.

* You can contribute and consume content with less effort.

If there are so many benefits to publishing, why are so few nurses doing it?

With every opportunity, there is a cost. One reason many nurses do not publish or participate in traditional forms of research relates to the barriers involved in the process. Take writing an article for a research journal as an example. Oermann and Hays (2002) identify four potential barriers:

* Lack of understanding of how to write for publication

* Writer's block

* Lack of time

* Fear of rejection

Reading this list, you might easily be able to add what prevents you from publishing (see Figure 7.1).

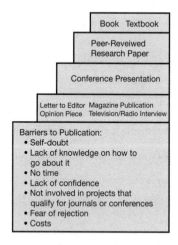

Figure 7.1: Traditional publishing presents large barriers to overcome.

With traditional publishing, the learning curve is fairly steep. Not only does it require specialized knowledge and experience, but your lack of control over what is published in the end leaves you feeling powerless. You can dedicate a lot of time and energy to writing, but if an article is rejected by a journal, it can be very discouraging. The option is always there to edit and revise, but that requires even more time, which many people can't afford to spend.

Doesn't social media content create more learning barriers?

There will always be a learning curve when you launch a new endeavor, and beginning to use social media is no exception. But, social media tools lower many of the barriers associated with traditional publishing. In fact, using social media to publish and share content can even enable you to overcome barriers and gain a foothold in traditional publishing (see Figure 7.2).

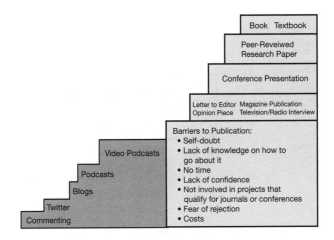

Figure 7.2: Social media lowers barriers and can even be a platform to publish in more traditional ways.

Perhaps David Eaves, an advocate of open and transparent government in Canada, best summarizes this philosophy by noting on his blog, "If writing is a muscle, this is my gym." Even though social media may involve a learning curve, the skills you gain enable you to develop your ability to communicate and share your expertise online, without the risk of wasted effort due to rejection.

This seems so fragmented. How does it all fit together?

The social media landscape is indeed complex, but learning about the tools will help you pull it all together.

Think about a celebrity. You might remember her from a movie, but you also see clips of her on television, radio, magazines, and newspapers. Regardless of where you see that celebrity, publicity builds her reputation. This is also true in less glamorous careers. The key is to link your efforts together; that way, your reputation builds. If you have a distributed presence, you can make an impact in a lot of places. By pulling those pieces together, you can build on what you have done (see Figure 7.3).

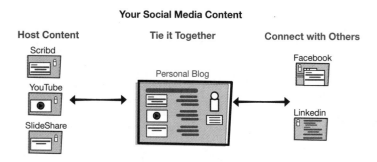

Figure 7.3: Publishing a blog is one way to centralize everything you're involved in.

How do you get started?

As a nurse, you have spent hours in classrooms and hospitals building a wealth of professional knowledge, which is often not shared with the public. How do you start sharing that knowledge? Here are a few ideas:

* Commenting

* Uploading content you have already created

* Experimenting with a blog

* Sharing information on Twitter

What are the benefits of commenting?

Commenting creates benefits for everyone. First, when you comment on content you find online, it helps you by building links to your profile. Second, commenting on content provides feedback, which helps the author of that content. Third, you help others by sharing your knowledge. When nurses begin to comment online, it changes how they share information. It's no longer simply about one person publishing his or her research, thoughts, or opinions; it becomes a continual dialogue that builds on itself.

TIP

Comments are one easy way to share your knowledge and awareness online.

What are the benefits of uploading content you have already created?

Over the course of your career, you may have developed articles, papers, presentations, or even audio and video materials. Surely others would benefit from having access to them! Offering these materials online is an excellent way to share your knowledge and thereby build your reputation. Choose the materials you want to share; then decide which sites will be the best place to share them, create accounts as needed, and spend time uploading your materials. (If you're not sure which web services handle what types of content, Table 7.1 contains a cheat sheet.)

7.1 Where you can upload your content

File Type	Web Service
Video	YouTube (http://www.youtube.com), blip.tv (http://blip.tv), Vimeo (http://vimeo.com)
Presentations (PowerPoint)	SlideShare (http://slideshare.com)

File Type	Web Service
Documents (Word files, PDFs, etc.)	Scribd (http://www.scribd.com)
Audio (podcasts)	Podomatic (http://www.podomatic.com)

What are the benefits of blogging?

As you will learn later in this chapter, a blog is not a blog anymore. Blogs are becoming much more powerful than simple journals on steroids. Blogging services such as WordPress give you the power to really manage your content. There is no single perfect use for a blog. In the nursing community alone, blogs are used in the following ways:

* To share life stories and build a support network, as with the blog "Head Nurse" (http://head-nurse.blogspot.com)

* To post useful resources such as research articles, as with the blog "Nursing Research: Show Me the Evidence" (http://evidencebasednursing.blogspot.com)

* To share video interviews of nursing leaders and researchers, as on the blog "Nursing Ideas" (http://nursingideas.ca)

These blogs differ in how they are useful for the author as well as how they are useful for the audience. Learning to use a blog to write a journal may seem like a pointless exercise, but consider what painfully tracing out every letter of the alphabet led to: your ability to write by hand. If you want to learn the tools, you have to practice using them.

What are the benefits of Twitter?

If you can write a sentence and use the cut-and-paste function on your computer, you can use Twitter. It's low maintenance, and there are no rules on how best to use it. (You'll find more on Twitter later in this chapter, including coverage of how to get started and some basic strategies on how to use it.) From detailing what you are working on (omitting patient information, of course) to sharing articles worth reading, Twitter has an endless number of uses.

For those of you who are still skeptics, this book is living proof of the serendipitous outcomes that can result when using Twitter, and I can point to a lot more. Connecting with others and sharing your interests and passions can have all sorts of great outcomes, which you often cannot plan!

Insights & Inspiration

Paul Bond, RN, CEN, MSN, ALNC

paul@paulbondRN

http://www.paulbond.com

I see the Internet as the ultimate equalizer in terms of information delivery. Nurses can update their knowledge or use new tools to share their expertise without disrupting their schedule. Nurses can create content that reaches wider audiences than traditional methods, and they can easily share what they are learning while keeping themselves up to date.

After sitting through numerous lectures and reading multiple books year after year to earn my continuing education credit, I thought there must be a better way to stay up to date. Because I have been an educator for much of my career, I began looking at ways to use social media to create content for nurses. Seeing podcasting as one option, I created "Emergency Nursing Today," a show produced every other week to share news and research relevant to emergency medical professionals. I also began PhoenixCE so that nurses and other health care professionals could update their knowledge and skills and earn continuing education credits. The content I created gives nurses the flexibility to easily stay up to date with news and research or earn their continuing education credits at their convenience.

Lesson: Begin a blog and talk about your passion. Search the Internet and see what else is out there. Connect with others who share your passion, find out what they need or want, and create content that serves them.

Blogging Basics

What is a blog?

A blog is a tool for sharing content. The name comes from the term Web log, a forum for regularly posting content. With blogs, you create a new post for each entry, enabling you to click the different entries much as you flip through pages in a book. The subject matter covered in blogs can be wildly different, ranging from specific topics to daily life events.

How have blogs evolved to become more useful?

Imagine a binder, to which you can easily add a new piece of paper. This is essentially how blogs behaved. The only problem was that content was organized by the date on which it was created—which is not always a practical or particularly useful way to organize information. As time passed, there was simply too much information to navigate easily, especially if you couldn't remember the month, date, or year in which a certain piece of information was created.

To deal with this, blogs have evolved to allow you to organize content in different ways and around different purposes. This turns what was traditionally thought of as an interesting hobby into an online content-management system. No longer just an online journal of sorts, a blog can serve as a platform for any purpose the author can envision.

How can you organize content?

A couple of basic ways to organize content improve on the traditional content-by-date model:

* Using categories
* Using tags

In addition, most blogs also offer some search functionality. This is extremely helpful, enabling you to locate information on other blogs easily, and helping visitors to your blog find what they are looking for.

How do you use categories to organize content?

Categories are core themes that you regularly plan to write about on your blog. They're like the sections you add to a binder at the beginning of each semester of school—one for each area of study, to enable you to quickly find the materials you need. For example, if you regularly write about a particular area of nursing, such as pediatric nursing, you might create a category for that topic on your blog. You might also create categories for professional issues, research news, work-related posts, and so on. When you create a category, people visiting your blog can easily see the topics on which you regularly post. They can then click a category to see all articles published in that category. Note that some posts may fit into multiple categories. For example, a post giving advice on preparing for a job interview might fit into both the "Advice for Student Nurses" and "Emergency Nursing" categories.

TIP

Decide what topics you plan to write about regularly, and create a category for each one.

How do you use tags to organize content?

Tags are labels that you can apply to a post. Tagging a post is like attaching a sticky note or creating an index of a specific topic or subject that is covered. Tagging a post attaches descriptive words, making it easy for others to locate content relating to those words. This improves users' ability to search your blog or to sort content. Some websites create tag clouds, which are aggregations of all the tags used on the site, with more commonly used tags appearing larger. This gives readers a way to see what type of content is talked about and the ability to click on a descriptor to see all the posts related to it.

TIP

If you use a tag very frequently, consider creating a new category for it.

What do you need to know to get started?

Creating a blog is not too complicated. You can do it in a few easy steps:

* Choose a blogging service—Most blogging services offer the same basic functionality, so browse around a bit and pick one you like. I'm biased toward WordPress (http://wordpress.com); it's known for regularly improving its service and adding new and useful features.

* Create an account—Creating an account is quick and simple. In addition to entering your information, you must validate your e-mail account. Remember to use your personal e-mail account unless you are creating the blog with specific permission from your work.

* Name your blog—When you sign up, you should have some idea of what you want to call your blog. If it is a personal blog, try using your name or the user name you employ for other social media sites. If you have a topic in mind, try to give it a fitting title—and remember, shorter is better. Note that your blogging service will use this name in the URL it creates for your blog.

* Create an About page—After you create your blog, the first page you should create is your About page. WordPress provides a default template, which you can edit as you see fit. The About page should indicate who you are and provide some explanation of what you want to do with your blog. For example, take a look at Nursing Influence's About page, http://nursinginfluence. com/about; it does not have to be fancy, just to the point.

* Choose your disclaimer—Better to be safe than sorry. Professionalism is important, as was covered in Chapter 3, and starting off on the right foot is the best way to avoid any problems in the future. Visit HONcode (http://www.hon.ch) or the Healthcare Blogger Code of Ethics website (http:// medbloggercode.com) to see guidelines and examples. You can also view other nursing blogs to see if they have examples you can use.

What features do you need to know?

Large books have been written on how to use all the blog tools. Following is a condensed version of what you need to understand to get started:

* Front end versus back end

* The anatomy of a blog

* The difference between posts and pages

How do I begin to make changes to my blog?

If you type the URL for your blog, it will bring you to your site, which everyone can see. This is called the blog's front end (see Figure 7.4). You must log in to the back end, shown in Figure 7.5, to edit or add content.

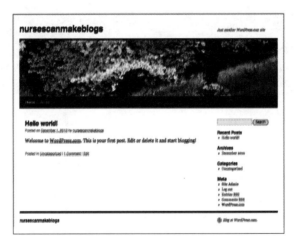

Figure 7.4: All blogs start out as blank templates; fortunately, it is easy to make the blog your own.

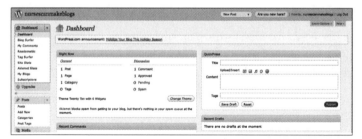

Figure 7.5: Wordpress gives you a clean back-end dashboard to control your blog.

What parts of the blog can I edit?

A blog contains the following elements (see Figure 7.6):

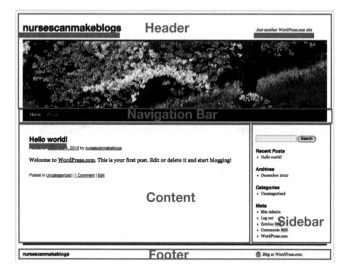

Figure 7.6: Blogs are made up of smaller parts that you can change to
personalize your site.

* Header—The header usually contains the blog's title, a tagline,
and an image or logo. Each blog comes with a basic default
heading, which you can change from the back end.

* Navigation menu—More sophisticated blogs automatically create a menu you can use to find important information. In WordPress, these are called pages. They contain content that is likely to stay the same over time, and that you do not want to be buried by newer content. Examples include your About page and your disclaimer.

* Content—The main content of a blog is the latest article, also called a post.

* Sidebar—Blogging services generally offer different themes—aesthetic layouts with relatively similar functionality. The placement of a sidebar will vary depending on the theme. They can appear on either side of the blog's content and may consist of multiple columns. These columns may contain information, such as categories, but may also have titles of recent posts or other features. Sidebars make it easier for visitors to navigate your blog.

* Footer—This is the area along the bottom of the blog. Some themes enable you to modify the footer and add more information or navigation features, such as recent posts or categories.

What is the difference between a post and a page?

Understanding the difference between a page and a post might be a bit confusing at first. When you look at them, they may seem very similar. Posts are the articles you write for your blog. As you write more articles, the newer ones will appear above the older ones. Pages are the areas on your blog where you keep important information that you want your readers to be able to access easily at any time. Information on pages won't get buried by new articles over time. You should put information that you want every visitor to find easily on a page; that way,

TIP

Create a new post for time-relevant content. Create a page for more permanent information.

it's only a click away, regardless of what post appears on the blog's main screen.

Once you understand the difference between posts and pages, it becomes easier to think about when you want to add a new page versus a new post. Adding new pages and posts is quite easy to do; WordPress does a nice job of keeping them separate.

What are some easy ways to improve your posts?

The best way to improve your content is to learn what tools are available to you. Most blogging services give you two ways to edit content. In the WordPress back end, beginners will use the WYSI-WYG (short for "what you see is what you get") Visual editor 99.9% of the time. Using the Visual editor toolbar, shown in Figure 7.7, you can do a lot of easy, yet important, tasks such as the following:

* Make headings bold—This helps users easily follow what you are writing about and quickly identify the next section.

* Create lists—Using bullets or numbers to create lists is an easy feature to use to improve your content and make reading easier.

* Upload and insert pictures—Text is great, but a picture really is worth a thousand words. Images can make a page more appealing, complement your content, or illustrate your point

* Create links—Links are the power of the Internet. With them, you don't have to cite a reference in name only; you can easily create a link to its website. When referring to a news article or research, you can help readers find that content by linking to it.

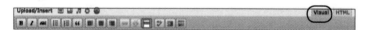

Figure 7.7: Switching between your Visual editor and HTML editor only takes a simple click.

Another way to add a little zip to a post is to embed content. This requires performing a simple copy-and-paste function, with a few extra clicks. When you embed content, you do more than just provide a link to that content—for example, a video or presentation. Instead, you actually include that content in your post. Here's a quick explanation of how to embed content in WordPress:

1. Find the content you want to embed. In this example, find a video you want to share on YouTube.

2. In YouTube, click the Embed button, select the code for the item you want to embed, right-click and copy it (see Figure 7.8).

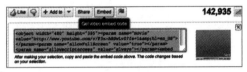

Figure 7.8: Content sites often offer the option to embed content on your blog by copying the code.

3. In the WordPress back end, open the post where you want to insert the clip.

4. Click the HTML tab on the right-hand corner of the page to switch to the HTML editor.

5. Right-click and select "Paste" to enter the code into the editor. If you already have started writing your post, you can decide where to place the content by pasting it before or after the code that is already there.

6. Click the Visual tab to change back to the Visual editor. Notice that a placeholder for the embedded content appears, so you know there is content there.

You're done! Now you can simply type what you want. When you publish your post, it will contain the video you embedded!

Most (if not all) content-sharing sites support embedding. Whenever you find content that you want to share, see if you can embed it on your website. This improves your content and helps share the content of the original author.

Twitter

What is Twitter?

Twitter is a microblogging service—a web service that lets you share status updates that contain 140 characters or less (letters, numbers, and spaces). The original question posed by Twitter was, "What are you doing?" A simple question, to be sure—but when you can easily share what you are doing, it allows for all sorts of possibilities!

What can you do with Twitter?

Twitter is a powerful tool because it functions with a firm rule—only 140 characters—and lets users run wild with it. Phil Baumann (2009), a nurse from Philadelphia, created a free ebook titled 140 Health Care Uses for Social Media. His ideas range from using social media to share daily health tips from authoritative sources to providing smoking cessation assistance, and from tracking disease-specific trends to tracking the safety and efficacy of pharmaceuticals—which, incidentally, has now been done (Rizo, Deshpande, Ing, & Seeman, 2010). This is not to suggest that you need to start using Twitter to do all those things, but it is important to recognize that Twitter has a lot of potential. To start, you can use Twitter to spread your knowledge and expertise by sharing articles or information related to what you are doing. Chapter 9 gets into more detail about how you can use Twitter to build your network.

How do you use Twitter?

It may sound strange, but one of the nice things about Twitter is its minimal functionality. As mentioned, you're limited to using 140 characters. In addition, there are a few tools you can use on Twitter, all of which can be found in a good tweet (see Figure 7.9):

* Mentions (@STTIpub)—Mentioning another Twitter user enables you to direct a tweet to that person. This alerts the person of your tweet, along with anyone who "follows" that person on Twitter.

* Hashtags (#nurses)—Tagging a tweet with a hashtag adds a descriptor to your tweet. This enables others searching for tweets on that topic to find your tweet.

* Links (http://su.pr/1ecPJV)—These direct others to a website, so you can share articles and other content. Note that some URLs exceed Twitter's 140-character limit; in this case, you can shorten links using services such as bit.ly (http://bit.ly) or Su.pr (http://su.pr).

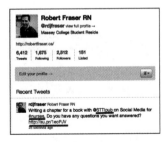

Figure 7.9: To use Twitter more effectively, consider how you can use one or more basic functions in your updates.

How do you get started?

With Twitter, it takes only a few minutes to sign up and start tweeting. You can start with something as simple as "Reading Nurse's Social Media Advantage." To get off the ground running, you just need to do the following:

* Create a Twitter account and user name.

* Fill in the biography and upload a picture.

* Enter your first tweet and click Send.

Frequently Asked Questions

 How do nurses find time to update these sites?

Everyone is a bit different, and that is perfectly acceptable. You do not have to update these sites on the hour. Finding a schedule that works for you will take a bit of practice. Just like going to the gym or setting aside time to study, individuals have certain patterns that work best for them. The best way to help others understand how you plan to use your social media accounts is to add information to that effect to your profile or About page. If you explain that you plan to post monthly updates, then people will know to check in monthly and can act accordingly. When learning to use these tools, be easy on yourself. Decide how they work best for you, and adjust your plan to use them accordingly.

 How can you push any meaningful information out in 140 characters?

One of the difficulties with Twitter is the limit. It can be very challenging to fit what you want to say into such a limited space. That being said, one could make the case that this limitation is also a benefit. It forces you to really consider what you want to share. Using Twitter becomes an art in the minimal. Instead of explaining everything you liked about a research paper or speech at a conference, you're limited to merely sharing a bit of basic information and a link to the content in question. If you want to submit a treatise on it, use your blog. If you feel compelled to write a response to an article beyond a simple recommendation, you need to know what tool to use.

 Where are the best online tutorials for getting started?

Everyone has an opinion, which is one of the benefits of using social media. If you are curious about how to do something with your blog or Twitter, you often can search your way toward an answer. YouTube has a lot of video tutorials, and

Google can help you find a fair number of articles on starting a blog or beginning to use Twitter. Whenever you have questions, using a search engine is a great way to find answers.

What kinds of applications make it easier to keep up with Twitter?

There are a number of ways you can make Twitter easier to use. For example, installing a browser extension (see Chapter 4 for a refresher on how to do this) such as Sharaholic enables you to simply click a button to share a link to a web page using social media services. There are also free desktop applications such as TweetDeck (http://tweetdeck.com) that enable you to type in messages instead of having to visit the Twitter web-site every time you want to tweet. And, if you have a smart phone, there are also a number of free applications that you can use to update Twitter and share pictures on the go.

How can you participate in Twitter without unwanted e-mails filling up your inbox?

One of the benefits of using Twitter is that you can update others and vice-versa without sending each other text messages or e-mails. However, most social media services want you to visit their site, so they will send you e-mail notifications. Feel free to turn those notifications off, which you can do at http://twitter.com/settings/notifications. Twitter should be a tool that empowers you, not enslaves you. You need to find how it fits into your schedule, not the other way around.

Should you Twitter or blog from work?

The answer to this question depends on your employer's perspectives on the technology. Your break times are technically your own, so if you have a mobile phone or Internet access, there is nothing to stop you from updating while you are at work. Remember, however, that while on the clock at work, you need to follow your employer's policies. If there is any chance it might come back to bite you, don't do it. Updating your status or writing one more blog post just isn't worth it. If you don't have your organization's blessing, wait until you get home.

Exercises

1. It's time to set up a space to share what you are doing by creating a social media account. When starting any new social media account, it's helpful to look at what others have done, to decide if you might want to imitate or improve on it. Start by searching WordPress or Twitter for the keyword "nurses."

2. Evaluate what other nurses are posting. Ask yourself: Does it look professional? Does it demonstrate their expertise? Are they doing things that you think are useful? Are they doing things you think are a waste of time? Learn from what you see.

3. Browse a few different blog services and choose the one you want to use. Then choose a user name and create your account.

4. Complete your About page and disclaimer, and submit your first post.

5. Ask others for feedback, and then submit a second post.

8

✳

Creating Quality Content

Do you:

Have ideas about what might be useful to post?

Know what form of content you naturally gravitate toward?

Have a strategy for creating new content?

Take small steps to improve the content you are making?

After you discover what social media tools are available, you must decide which tools are best for you. Then, when you get the hang of using them, you can work toward improving the quality of your content. No one is perfect in the beginning! Right out of the gate, you should look for ways to improve.

Quality is never an accident; it is always the result of high intention, sincere effort, intelligent direction, and skillful execution; it represents the wise choice of many alternatives."

–William A. Foster

Improve Your Work

Why do you need to focus on quality?

Many people blog, post status updates, or send tweets just to get things off their chest. It's a little like therapy. But with social media, there is a second person involved: the person who takes that message in. In the beginning, it's fine to focus on using social media for your own benefit. But, if you want to use social media to bolster your reputation, you need to think about how you can improve your content to make it useful to others. Social media may not yet be as highly regarded as more traditional types of publication (magazine articles or research journals), but that does not mean quality is unimportant in the social media realm. Here are just a few reasons to focus on quality:

* Quality content makes your message more clear to your audience.

* It saves your reader or viewer from dealing with time-consuming content.

* It reflects your attention to detail.

* It may be used as part of your portfolio.

* Improving the quality of your posts enables others to see your progression.

* It helps you build the reputation of nurses with the public and other professionals.

* It forces you to think critically and reflect on the reasons for your opinions.

How good does your content have to be?

This is a bit of a gray area. Of course, there is no standard when it comes to participating in social media. Anyone can contribute. But as nurses, we automatically assume an elevated position of authority. That means we should take responsibility to post quality content, and we must stand behind what we post. You don't have to lose sleep over the quality of your posts, but you should take some pride in what you produce. Remember, with social media, you have an opportunity to develop—a process that can take some time. As an added bonus, learning to clearly and concisely express your thoughts and defend your position in social media can translate to the way you speak in the workplace or write for assignments at work or school or for fun.

TIP

Don't let the need for perfection stop you from starting!

What should you try to improve first?

When you have a solid understanding of the differences among the various social media sites and the services they offer, think about what form of content you prefer to create. Using social media isn't something that you are being forced to do, so why not choose the type of content you prefer, or even like, to create? In general, your choices are as follows:

* Text—Some people have a natural talent for writing, and others, well, don't. If you like to express yourself by writing down your thoughts or ideas, then play to this strength by blogging, microblogging, using document hosts to upload Word documents and PDF files, or even using a site such as Xtranormal (http://www.xtranormal.com), a website that creates animated movies from scripts you submit. Even if you struggle with writing, there may be some merit to using text-oriented social media tools. Forcing yourself to write short pieces on your ideas will not only help you develop this essential skill, it might also help you learn to love writing.

* Audio—Individuals who prefer to talk about their ideas may feel more comfortable using audio recordings to communicate their thoughts—for example, creating their own podcast using PodOmatic (http://www.podomatic.com). Even if you don't like speaking in front of crowds, developing audio content to go with your written work may help you to improve your public speaking—something that will be helpful if you ever need to give a presentation for work.

* Visual—If you wish, you can present your ideas in a more visual way, whether it's posting diagrams or images on Flickr (http://www.flickr.com), posting a PowerPoint presentation on SlideShare (http://www.slideshare.net), or using a service such as Animoto (http://animoto.com) or Prezi (http://prezi.com) to create a video slideshow on the Internet. Posting videos, from animations to interviews, on sites such as YouTube (http://www.youtube.com) is another great option for sharing ideas online.

How do you build on these skill sets?

If you're just getting started, there are many ways to improve your skill sets, such as:

* Practice and practice more.

* Edit and revise your old work to look for ways to develop it further.

* Ask if you can create materials for your employer.

Even if you consider yourself to be more accomplished—say, you're a strong writer, or you're experienced with public speaking—you can build your skills by pushing yourself into new areas. Using multiple modes of media to express your ideas will improve your ability to communicate, as well as enable others to choose which format is best for them. For example, even if you consider yourself a writer, creating a series of great slides might help a visual thinker to really grasp what you are trying to communicate. The more formats you develop, the wider your audience becomes and the more effectively you can teach others.

Identifying Your Audience

Why does making quality content matter, if no one is listening?

Why assume no one is listening? Thankfully, search engines have made it possible to find and hear anyone who is producing content. Improving the quality of your content makes it more likely that search engines will find it. This is because better content increases the likelihood others will link to your site, and quality of the content impacts search ranking.

Remember, social media is not just about pushing content out. The second component of social media is participation. When people read your comments on other sites, they are more likely to follow your links to see what you are producing. If the content you produce is useful, others are likely to share links to your website, because it is a resource that they can pass on to their own network.

How do you know what your audience wants?

To understand what people want, you have to understand them. The best way to do that is to ask them, and to really listen to their response. Then, watch to see what they do.

Participating in online communities can enable you to find your target audience. It gives you a chance to get to know them and to ask them what types of resources would be useful for them.

This research does not even have to be online. Try talking to family, friends, or other people you know who might be in your target audience. Then try searching the different web services. See if you can find any traces of the content you are thinking about making. Ask yourself these questions:

* Is anyone else out there producing this content?

* Are there any examples of where this has been successful?

* If no one has tried this before, why not?

    * Do I have an original idea, or something that just cannot work?

    * How can I get my audience to pay attention, if they are not already?

Critically thinking about your plans for content can help you investigate what is happening online, think about how you can be original, and prevent you from trying to invent a square wheel.

How do you develop an audience?

When it comes to developing an audience, it seems people often err in one of two ways: by underplanning or by overplanning.

Some people prefer to fly by the seat of their pants. Although that may work, it can backfire, putting you somewhere you don't want to be. On the other end of the spectrum is overplanning: spending too much time strategizing. This can be terribly frustrating if your audience does not develop or if the wrong people like your content.

The key is to develop a balance between underplanning and overplanning. Consider whom you want to benefit. Perhaps you want to provide advice for mid-career nurses about saving for retirement. Or maybe you want to share tips with new nurses about surviving their first job. If you think about the people you are creating content for, you can experiment. Produce content for that group and see what sticks; then keep doing what works.

Here are some additional ideas for growing your audience:

1. Give it time—Don't feel frustrated after a week, month, or even a year if you haven't gained a huge following. Developing an audience takes time, and there's no way to rush things.

2. Focus on content—Keep producing content. Generating new content and improving the content you produce are important. Developing more resources means more people will find your site, due to search engines, and increases the likelihood they will stay. Never neglect producing content in an attempt to find your audience.

3. Share links—Links play an important part in how your content ranks in the search engine. Putting links in your blog posts can help demonstrate that you are providing useful resources. Also, when others link to you, it shows you have created a useful resource.

4. Join other online conversations—Find discussion boards, blogs, and other sites that discuss content online. Don't start by linking to your content; instead, start by participating and helping others. When they click to find your information, they will learn about what you are doing.

5. Change your e-mail signature—Adding a link to your online projects in your e-mail signature is another way to get traffic. It is a subtle way to let your acquaintances know what you are doing online, and a good way for new contacts to find out more about you.

6. Promote your subscription options—No matter what content you produce, remind people where and how they can find out more. If you offer a way to subscribe to e-mails, remind users to subscribe. Some users might not know about your offerings, and other users might not sign up if you do not ask them. Not everyone will sign up, but asking cannot hurt your chances.

7. Go offline—Remember, social media is just a tool. It doesn't require you to be on your computer 24/7. Putting up a flyer on a bulletin board and mentioning your site to others at a conference are great ways to promote your work. Don't simply say, "Go to my website!" for no reason. Instead, try to bring it up when it relates to the conversation. Say, "You might find my [video, podcast, blog] on this topic useful," or, "I have actually produced a few posts about [insert topic]."

Brainstorming

What should you do first?

There is no textbook to tell you the right or wrong answers for what type of content you should create. When you have a topic and a potential audience in mind, it's time to get creative. Fortunately, nurses have a long history of being creative when it comes to solving patient problems; now's your chance to be creative with producing content. You don't have to come up with a new unified theory of nursing. Instead, try to think of some core pieces of information that would be useful, as well as lighter pieces of information such as latest or related research and news.

What are other people doing?

Any online search will bring up all sorts of content produced by nurses. There are too many to list all of them, but here are examples of ideas that nurses have had for using social media:

* *Evidence-Based Nursing* blog (http://evidencebasednursing. blogspot.com)—This blog provides monthly updates of useful research articles for nurses.

* *How to Be a Nurse* ebook (available from http://impacted-nurse.com)—This PDF, made by a nurse from Australia, is a comical and practical guide for nursing students. It's part of a series of resources on his ironically named site, "Impacted Nurse."

* *Confessions of a Nursing Student* (http://www.youtube.com/user/hannahdemarco)—Hannah Demarco made a video journal of what she was learning and experiencing in nursing school. Her videos have received more than 200,000 views.

* *Nursing Students on the Future of Nursing Report* (http://inqri.blogspot.com/2010/11/nursing-students-on-future-of-nursing.html)—Professor Terri Schmitt's informatics class wrote a blog post responding to a report on the future of nursing by the Institute of Medicine.

* *Nursing Informatics Competencies: Self Assessment for Nurses* (http://www.slideshare.net/junek/nursing-informatics-competencies-self-assessment-for-nurses)—Nurse June Kaminski posted her presentation for a nursing conference online. It has since been viewed more than 2,000 times.

* *Drawing on Experience* (http://wilomis.wordpress.com/2010/12/04/attn-nurses-i-need-your-help)—New graduate Will Hardy's blog includes his thoughts on nursing, along with cartoons he draws. In one post, he asked experienced nurses for advice for his first job, which received a large response.

These are just a few ideas. The possibilities are limited only by your creativity and your willingness to learn to produce new forms of content.

Insights & Inspiration

Jamie Davis, BA, RN, EMT-P

@podmedic

http://podmedic.com

I started podcasting while looking for a resource providing regular updates on the world of nursing and patient care. When I found there was no such resource for nurses, I created a show of my own. I now have five weekly podcasts, including shows for paramedics, nurses, and other health professionals. With more than 2 million episode downloads delivered, I am able to share recent health news, discussions, and commentary with people around the world.

My original radio-style shows have evolved to include video versions, while my career has evolved into a full-time health care journalist and social media consultant. In 2008, I realized there was no resource to collate online medical radio and TV programs. I started the ProMedNetwork.com site to provide a single location for high-quality, online medical and health programming.

Lesson: Each one of us has valuable experiences to share with other health professionals and patients. There can never be too many shows in any topic area. The audience will follow the content.

How can you keep track of your ideas?

Once you develop the courage to be creative with social media content, you'll start to have ideas all the time. This can be a blessing and a curse. You might not have time to write "Ten Tips for Nursing Students During a Code" when the idea strikes you during a code! It's critical that you develop a system to remember your ideas. That way, when you have time, you don't sit there trying to think of what content to produce. A few easy ways are to write yourself a note, send yourself an e-mail, or make a quick draft post for your blog (see Figure 8.1).

TIP

There are great podcasts on almost any topic, produced each week by people just like you.

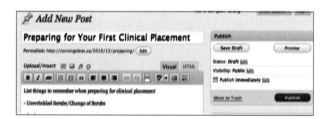

Figure 8.1: Blogs let you create draft posts, which can be a great way to track ideas you want to write about.

Continually Improving Content

How do you make your content successful?

Here are a few ideas to keep in mind:

* Develop a clear purpose—If you are planning any type of series or content, develop a clear focus. A white paper with blogging tips will not be used if people don't know what it is

for. Similarly nurses will not check back every week to your news podcast if they don't know what you are doing. For all the content you create, try to have a clear focus—although you should feel free to have different spaces for different things. Many nurses have one blog they use for journaling and another where they place content focused on a single issue (research, infusion nursing, staff development, global health, etc.).

* Be sensitive to time—Time is valuable to everyone. You might be giving content away free of charge, but if you require your users to spend a lot of time to access it, they may still view the cost as too high. There is no golden rule for how long a blog post or video should be, but you should always ask yourself whether you are being as concise as possible. Twitter is nice in this respect because it forces you to say something short, such as "This is a great article and worth reading." After all, you don't need to re-write the entire article, even if you have the space to do so! That being said, if you feel you have a big idea, there is nothing wrong with writing a long post with your views. Just make sure you are respectful of users' time and that you are providing them with value.

* Save users time—This is a slightly different rule in the sense that whenever you can share a way to save users' time, you will develop a loyal audience. For example, gathering the latest on diabetes research or wound care takes time. If you can provide content that helps others save time, you will provide a useful resource people will come to appreciate.

* Have a consistent release schedule—If you want to keep your audience coming back, they need to know when to check. Visiting a channel only to find it hasn't been updated can be frustrating. If users know to check back once a month, however, their expectations will be in check. A "weekly" news site for nurses that updates only once a month or very irregularly will be less successful than one that is reliably updated. It is better to post less often and more consistently than frequently and irregularly.

✳ Provide resource or reference material—Always provide links, if possible, and references to your sources. Even with videos, posting links or references allows users to check the primary source and learn more about issues you might briefly mention.

✳ Provide value—Creating content that teaches, explains, or helps users to learn how to do something builds trust and loyalty. Think about mentors and teachers who have made the biggest impact on you. They are the ones who took time to help you understand content. If you can help others to learn difficult-to-understand concepts, or can provide unique insight or experience, it will help others to learn. That is something they will value!

✳ Support interaction and feedback—Learn from traditional media. Many talk-show hosts interact with the audience between commercials as well as before and after the show. Developing relationships with your audience helps your audience feel listened to and appreciated. It also helps you to learn what they think. Take their thoughts into account as you develop your content. In addition to helping you improve your content, it will help assure your audience that you are listening.

What are some easy ways to improve your blog content?

Here are a few ways to improve your blog content:

✳ Spell-check and edit—Dollar for dollar—really, minute for minute—this is the best investment you can make in your content. It might be hard to find the time, but a second or third read of your content can help you to catch spelling mistakes or incorrect grammar. This is the simplest way to make your content better.

✳ Make it useful—Ask yourself, What is the point? If you don't know, then your readers won't either. Whether writing a reaction or opinion, focus your thoughts to come up with a point that you want to get across. Your content can be educational or informative, can raise another perspective, can add new information, or can highlight useful resources. What should your reader remember? When should users tell others about this content?

* Make it unique—Following the lead of others is a good way to start, but you need to be different to stand out. Do it better, or differently. Do not simply copy and paste.

* Outline and summarize—Telling people what they can expect out of your content helps them identify whether it is what they are looking for. Summarizing helps them recap what they learned or should take away. Also, don't always feel you have to go on at length about issues. Providing bullet points can be very useful.

How do you make quality audio content?

Following are a few ways to make quality audio content. (Note that this advice relates to audio for video recordings, too.)

* Get a microphone—Listening to poor-quality audio is like reading a textbook written by hand on soiled paper. Indeed, poor-quality audio can make it difficult to concentrate on what is being said. Invest in a decent microphone!

* Learn to use your mic—Once you have your mic, practice using it. Test it to see how close or far you need to be to get clear sounds, without cracking or popping.

* Eliminate background noise—Pick a quiet room where you will not be interrupted or have to deal with distracting noises. Barking dogs and furnaces break listeners' concentration and prevent them from hearing your message.

TIP

Find a podcast you like and model your own show's design and flow after it.

* Format and edit—When making a series, try to keep it consistent.

Once you record it, take time to edit your recording to help polish it.

* Enunciate and use expression—Mumbling or using a monotone can prevent listeners from hearing what you are saying, or may result in their being too bored to keep listening. Practice pronouncing difficult words and using different tones to emphasize important parts and to help convey meaning.

How can video quality be improved?

Here are a few ways to make quality video content:

* Location, location, location—When you're on the go and want to record something, choose your location carefully. Make sure there is good lighting and minimal background noise.

* Sound matters—Video quality is important, but sound is more so. If there is no audio, there is no message—and no one will watch a video that has no meaning. Make sure you capture what is being said clearly so viewers can easily hear it.

* Framing—Zoom and focus on your subject. If you are far away, try to zoom in so that facial expressions and gestures are easy to make out. They convey a lot in the way of nonverbal communication.

* Avoid shadows—The camera makes things darker, so make sure your subject does not have shadows that obscure his or her face. Otherwise, you'll lose your subject's expression.

* Practice—Because video captures your speech and body language, you need to practice speaking clearly and controlling your movement. Mumbling and fidgeting will distract from the content.

* Edit—Through simple editing, you can remove unnecessary parts and mistakes. Editing also enables you to insert a title and credits and to include a link to your website. There are a number of tools for editing your video clips and countless video tutorials online to teach you how to use them.

"Life is a gift, and it offers us the privilege, opportunity, and responsibility to give something back by becoming more."

–Anthony Robbins

Frequently Asked Questions

 Can posting better-quality content help you get a job?

Anytime you develop yourself and demonstrate your commitment to helping others and producing high-quality work, it makes you a more valuable employee. Although your work in social media probably won't appear on your job application, what you learn from producing content—your creativity and your professionalism—is sure to come across, and it may well have an impact on your job search.

 How does quality content affect your career in the long run?

Spending time developing the quality of your content helps to firmly establish you as an expert on a subject. If you can convey your knowledge and experience effectively, it helps organizations and individuals seeking your skill sets to find you. This can translate into better job offers, opportunities to collaborate on research, or even work as a consultant in your area.

 What is the point of using different platforms to share the same idea?

The more ways you distribute your ideas and materials, the more ways others can discover them and find them useful. Just as people have different tastes and opinions, they tend to have preferences when it comes to learning. Think about how it was in school. Some people liked listening to a teacher; others needed to see the example drawn on the chalkboard; still others just wanted to read their textbook. The same is true on the Internet. Creating content for multiple platforms enables users to choose the format that works best for them. As an added bonus, by creating content for different platforms, you demonstrate that you have a lot of talent, are extremely considerate, and are dedicated to your cause.

 How can you prevent your voice from being lost?

Quality always rises to the top. It may take time, but persistence and getting involved with others will always trump production of mediocre content. Time is at a premium these days, and no one wastes it intentionally. If you make a lot of bad content, you will quickly lose your audience. If you produce quality content, even in small quantities, people will eventually find it and share it.

 Why put in the effort if no one takes social media seriously?

The proof is in the pudding: The Internet is clearly not going away. As health care organizations and health care leaders see the results of using social media, the ability to generate good content will become a more valued skill. Years ago, a nurse who could also perform research might not have been considered an asset. But, the shift to evidence-based care and the need to translate research change how we evaluate skill sets. Plus, developing your communication skills will never hurt your career. These skills are transferable; you can use them in many different ways to help an organization. Any time you invest in developing your computer literacy, your knowledge of the Internet, or your ability to create learning resources for others, it will pay off.

 What are the down sides to using certain types of content?

With every type of content, there is a cost-to-benefit ratio. Written content may involve the least in terms of overhead, but it can fail to convey the writer's tone and voice. Audio content might be more entertaining than written content, but it can be hard to follow when ideas are complex. And, while video format may have the most features, it is harder to find because no matter how long a video is, search engines can only see its title. When you are choosing what type of content to create, think about what might be beneficial or challenging for your audience. For example, if you are targeting nurses in rural areas, video might be too slow to download. In that case, a blog might be a more useful resource.

 What is the most effective way to get people to pay attention to an issue or raise awareness?

Unfortunately, there is no "secret sauce" or magical ingredient that I can give you. The best advice I have is to generate content that people care about, and then use all the time you can to interact with people, developing relationships and bringing awareness to your cause. Jennifer Aaker and Andy Smith (2010) propose you F+GET: focus, grab attention, engage, and take action.

Exercises

1. Improving the quality of content is really about focusing and being intentional about the content you create. One easy way to do this is to develop a rough plan. Yes, the plan might change, but creating a plan lets you test out new ideas and see how they work. A plan also helps you to move forward. Even if your direction changes, you will understand what works and be able to make small changes to accomplish new goals. To develop a plan, start by identifying your voice. Using the form at the end of this chapter, write your preferences for communicating in the left-most column. You can choose one or' two ways; write them down in order of preference.

2. In the form's second column, identify and write down what issues you are passionate about or want to specialize in.

3. Consider who you might be able to help or target with your content. There is no right answer; it's all about whom you

want to market your knowledge or services to. Write down your audience in the form's third column.

4. Get creative and make a list of things that you think would be interesting to make. Don't focus on what you think you can do; write what you would love to see in the fourth column of the form. Be bold!

5. Pick a place to start. In the form's fifth column, write down two or three forms of content you want to focus on creating. Then add a few more that you hope to learn how to do in the future.'

Hold on to this piece of paper; save it and use it. Give yourself a time line. Think about when you might realistically be able to accomplish some of these things, and try to set some goals for yourself.

Find your voice   List your passions   Identify your audience   What is possible?   Where can I start?   Goals

9

*

Building Your Online Network

Social media is made possible by web services. These are merely the tools that host media, however. The secret sauce of these tools is the people.

Social media brings people together and provides new ways to connect. Think about it: Even the highest quality textbook or video is not very valuable unless it has an audience. Similarly, having a Facebook or Twitter account is not very useful unless you utilize it for the purpose for which it was intended: to connect with people in new and meaningful ways.

"It is all about people. It is about networking and being nice to people and not burning any bridges."

                                                              --Mike Davidson

Social Networks

What are some of the advantages of social network sites over traditional address books?

Social network sites offer a number of advantages over traditional methods of organizing your contacts and keeping in touch with them. Traditional methods such as telephone books, directories, or even your own paper- or computer-based address book regularly go out of date. They only exist in one place, so if you don't have it with you, you're out of luck. Traditional methods are also separate from the mode of communication you use, meaning that just having someone's mailing address doesn't necessarily make it possible to call them or get in touch.

Social networks offer a new way to keep up to date with friends and colleagues. They offer a number of advantages:

* Their contact information is always up to date.

* More information—personal or professional interests, pictures, etc.—is available.

* Being connected enables you to receive additional information, such as status updates, posted pictures, or changes in employment.

* They offer you the ability to send messages, often with different formats (private/public, text, video, etc.).

* Participating in social networking can remind you to reconnect with old contacts.

* You can see people's connections to others.

How do social networks change traditional methods of networking?

You can use social networks in a number of ways. Even if you limit their use to a simple address-book replacement, they can be very beneficial for keeping in touch with your contacts. Additionally, social networks expose hidden connections and lower the barrier for developing your network. For example, in the old days, when you met a new coworker, it might have taken years for you to figure out that her cousin was your best friend in high school. Being able to find out that your college roommate happens to know the manager of the department you are applying to, or a professor at the university where you are considering applying for your doctorate of nursing practice (DNP), is incredibly valuable!

Another benefit is the ability to explore networks and build relationships. When you meet someone at a conference, you may get that person's contact information, but that doesn't give you the ability to look through a list of all of his or her connections. In the past, making such a request would have been considered ridiculous, rude, or both. Now, however, you have full license to explore networks and relationships. Adding others to your network on sites such as LinkedIn or Facebook enables you to see them and their contacts.

What types of social-networking tools are there for managing contacts?

Several types of social-networking tools are available for maintaining contacts, including the following:

* Online address books—These tools enable you to store your contact information online. One benefit of using an online address book is that you can access your information anywhere. Information is secure, and cannot be lost. With most of these services, you can also synchronize data to the address book

for your e-mail service or on your computer. One example of an online address book service is Plaxo (http://www.plaxo.com).

* Contact-management systems—These systems do more than just keep track of your contacts. They support relationship management. With these systems, you can find the latest news about your contacts, gleaned from their tweets, blog posts, and updates on various social media sites. These systems can also be set up to send timely reminders about when to get in touch with certain contacts. An example of a contact-management system is Gist (http://gist.com), which integrates with Gmail.

* Social networks—Sites such as Facebook (http://www.facebook.com) and LinkedIn (http://www.linkedin.com) provide online space to connect and interact with your contacts, enabling you to develop your relationships. Information about your contacts is updated by the individuals themselves.

These are the major social-networking tools for managing contacts, but really, any tool that enables you to keep up to date with a contact, as well as get in touch with that person, is a social-networking tool. Don't limit yourself to using only these types of tools to build and sustain relationships. Be creative! Any tool you can use to develop a relationship will be beneficial.

What steps are involved in managing and developing your contacts?

Just having an account with a web service and having a few contacts on it doesn't mean you have a strong network of relationships. To start building your relationships, you'll want to do the following:

* Initiate contact—Facebook and LinkedIn enable you to search for and add friends to your network, which is why they are considered more powerful social-networking tools than, say, online address books.

✳ Store contact information—This function is reason alone to create an online address book or use a contact-management system. There's no use in having a drawer full of business cards; at minimum, you need a way to organize and store your contacts and, if possible, a system to keep in touch with them on a regular basis.

✳ Update contact information—This is the danger of a neglected Rolodex: outdated contact information. If you aren't regularly in touch with your contacts, keeping their information up to date, you risk losing the ability to contact them at all.

✳ Sustain contact online and offline—Like plants, relationships need to be nurtured to grow. You need to find a way to keep in touch with your contacts, especially since you may go years between seeing them in person. This is one reason social-networking sites and contact-management services are useful: They provide you that healthy reminder to catch up with someone you have not seen in a while.

Does it matter if you don't have a lot of contacts when you start?

Developing a strong network takes time. Just as buying an address book doesn't mean you'll automatically have enough contacts to fill it, neither does creating an account online mean you'll automatically have loads of people in your network. By managing your contacts, however, you can develop a robust network over time. And of course, even if you're just getting started with social networking, you likely have at least some contacts you can add already. Be sure to add those contacts right from the beginning and add to them as you go. Over time, your network will grow. More importantly, you'll be able to develop those relationships, not just collect contact information.

TIP If you're mindful about using social-networking tools to develop relationships, over time, your network will grow.

Adding Contacts

How do you add contacts to an address book?

After you create an account with an online address book, you might be able to import contact information you've entered into your e-mail program or stored elsewhere on your computer. Beyond that, you should dedicate time to copying entries from any paper-based address books you've maintained over the years as well as from business cards you have collected.

When entering contact information, keep the following points in mind:

* Enter all the information you have: job titles, company, etc.

* Add any additional information you know, such as personal e-mail or home addresses.

* Enter other relevant details or information, such as where you met the person, any mutual acquaintances, or the person's specialty.

Hopefully, when you enter this information, you'll have a clear memory of who the person is—especially if you met recently. But, if you've forgotten who Dave Fennell, MBA, is, then having his contact information will not do you any good.

How do you add contacts to a contact-management system?

When you first create your account, you will need to import your contacts from your e-mail program or the address book you store on your computer. Next, you will need to set up your preferences and, if possible, integrate the contact-management system with your e-mail and calendar service. If you take time to integrate the service with your Gmail account, it will provide you with even more information while you go through your regular e-mail workflow (see Figure 9.1).

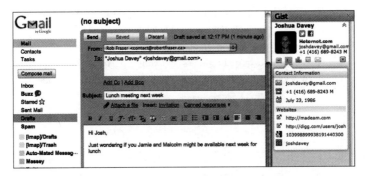

Figure 9.1: Using a content-management system in conjunction with Gmail provides an image and information of the person who sends you an e-mail to the right
of the message.

How do you add contacts to a social-networking site?

After you have set up your profile on a social-networking site, you
can begin to add people to your friends list or contacts list. These
services usually enable you to find people you know by importing
contact information from other services. The other option you have
is to manually add individuals by doing one of the following:

* Searching for their names—If you are looking for specific
  people, searching is one way to find them. It may be difficult
  if their name is a common one, but having additional details
  about them, such as their hometown, may help you find their
  profile.

* Searching friends' contacts—One great way to find friends is
  by looking at whom your existing connections have added.
  Although no one has the exact same set of contacts, you'll
  often find that family members have added other relatives
  you know, friends from school have found other classmates,
  and coworkers have already connected with other work colleagues.

* Seeing a link to their social networking profile—As social
  networks gain popularity, people have begun placing links
  to their profiles in e-mail signatures and on their websites.
  This tells you that the person is using a particular social-
  networking site, and you can reach out to him or her there.

Are there practices you need to avoid when adding people?

When participating in social networks, you're not just using online
tools; you're interacting with real people. It's important to remember how it feels to be on the other side of digital communication.
Think of social networking as being similar to interacting with others at a cocktail party or social gathering. It's OK to make a few
social faux pas, but if you cross the line too many times, you're not
going to build any meaningful relationships.

Here are a few things to keep in mind when you are adding new
contacts:

* Don't invite your entire contact list to join a social-networking
  site—No one feels special when they receive a generic e-mail
  that says "I have joined X site and think you should join too!"
  People are bombarded with e-mail and can tell the difference
  between a personal e-mail and a scripted one. A few people
  might join, but they are more likely to be annoyed.

* Don't send generic contact request messages to people you
  don't know very well—Although social network sites do offer
  prewritten invitations—"Hi [insert name here], I would like
  to [be friends/network with you] on [insert service name here].
  Thanks! [your name here]"—these messages sound automated
  and robotic. Indeed, they defeat the entire purpose of social
  networks: to build relationships. You would never walk up to
  someone and say, "Hi! May I have all your contact information and personal details? Thank you!" You might add some
  of your really close friends in this way without thinking too
  much about it, but the less well you know the person, the
  more you should avoid generic invites.

* Don't contact people you don't know personally without explaining why you want to connect—Social-networking sites enable you to find others with similar interests, specialties, or hobbies. But just having something in common doesn't mean that if you attempt to connect with a person, he or she will know that you want to connect because both of you are nurses or fans of Michael Jackson. Again, picture someone walking up to you, asking for your business card, and then walking away. It doesn't give a good first impression, and it doesn't give the person a good reason to accept your contact request.

* Don't contact a stranger for "potential future interest"—Asking a person for his or her name at a party "in case I want to talk to you later" seems laughable. You only need someone's name if you are being introduced to that person or if you are starting up a conversation. If you do not have any valid reason for contacting someone, you are wasting that person's time and yours. Having one more contact on Facebook and LinkedIn won't help you, and it wastes time you should be spending on relationships you do have.

* Do send a few personal e-mails—Think about people you know who might be interested in connecting with you online and take time to write a personal e-mail to request that they do so. Even if that person isn't interested, knowing you thought of him or her and believed he or she might find the site useful is likely to be appreciated. It can also be an excuse to enjoy an overdue conversation.

* Do make personal contact requests whenever possible—Take time to write a note when you request to add someone to a social network. It reminds people that they actually know you and that they should like you because you are a friendly person. Explain how you found them, that you recently thought about them and wanted to get back in touch, and that you wanted to extend the opportunity to reconnect through this social-networking site.

* Do explain why you want to add a person you do not know—Sending a message explaining that you both know Cynthia,

went to the same high school, or practice in the same specialty provides meaningful background information that helps the other person understand why you have initiated contact. This makes it far more likely that a person will accept your request.

* Do reach out to people you do not know with opportunities— Using a social-networking site to get in touch with people you do not know but might have reason to contact is perfectly acceptable. In your invitation, explain why you want to get in touch with that person and start a conversation. The person can evaluate your offer to connect and see the opportunity. It also invites the person to join a conversation, which invites a response rather than leaving the person with only two options: "accept" or "decline."

> *Import* means to copy information from one service to another. *Invite* means to use information from one service to invite your contacts to a new service.

How do you find people to network with online?

Keep these points in mind when looking for people to network with online:

* Identify shared interests and opportunities—Looking for people with shared interests and specialties is a great way to find useful connections. When you connect with others in your field, you can share resources and possibly collaborate in the future.

* Provide information and answer questions—Becoming a resource to others online is a great way to build your reputation and help others. It may often lead to further discussions and is a good way to build relationships.

* Find conversations and discussions to join—Through social networks, people can gather around topics of interest. You meet more people simply by participating in the conversation. When you get to know people through shared interests, you

can show your expertise or demonstrate interest in the area. When you find experts and others who are interested in a field, you can ask them for useful resources and recommendations or provide information for them.

* Utilize the search function—There is always the option to just try keywords in the web service's search engine. The search engine is a great tool to find others with common interests in their profiles or to locate groups discussing your interest. Looking for these keywords helps lead you to the right people; it is then up to you to start the conversation and build the relationship.

* Build a group or start a discussion—If you don't find others who are discussing your topic of interest, why not be the first to start that conversation? Being the first enables you to lead the discussion and is a great way to connect with others and develop your profile.

How often should you get in touch with your contacts?

When deciding how often to contact someone, ask yourself these questions:

* What is your relationship? A manager or boss may benefit from regular updates, even if they are not required. A director or colleague might need less contact. In that case, just "getting in touch" too often can be annoying.

* How much is too much? Think about how often you want people to contact you. At what frequency might you become a disturbance or be considered annoying? These online systems can help you keep in regular contact, but that doesn't mean you need to e-mail everyone every week.

* How much is too little? You don't want to go so long without touching base that people forget who you are! With some online tools, you can set reminders, so that if you haven't reached out in a while, you'll receive a reminder to do so.

Joining Communities

Are there rules for joining online conversations?

Some websites have guidelines for acceptable use. A great example is Mashable's (2010) guidelines, which offer eight easy principles:

* No personal attacks.

* Hate speech will not be tolerated.

* Language needs to respect others.

* Spam will be removed.

* Constructive criticism is allowed; smear tactics are not.

* Comments need to be relevant.

* Quality of conversation needs to be maintained.

* Every user needs to take part in building the community.

These rules can apply to any situation. Being kind and keeping comments respectful are the important points to remember. Constructive arguments and dialogue are encouraged; name-calling and insults are not.

Where are these online discussions taking place?

Conversations are happening in many different ways online. Social-networking sites such as LinkedIn and Facebook enable you to create groups and fan pages around special interests or for groups and associations. Taking time to search for your areas of expertise will usually result in finding people using these social-networking sites to meet others with shared interests.

Adding comments on news websites or blogs is another way to have conversations around a particular topic or interest. The original article is not the only thing you can respond to; you can also reply to other individuals' comments. Microblogs have created another way to follow conversations. Searching for a hashtag can help you find and follow a conversation, and others can find your comments there. One example is RNChat (http://rnchat.org), a regular discussion on Twitter about various nursing-related topics. Using Twitter's search functionality or Tweetchat (http://tweetchat.com), you can follow and participate in conversations with nurses from around the world.

What is the point of joining these conversations?

Taking part in online discussions is a great way to network and participate in sharing and developing ideas. Finding other nurses online is an excellent way to connect with others who are passionate about the same topics as you are. Through getting to know other nurses, you can share ideas, find support, and discover opportunities and new ways to work with others.

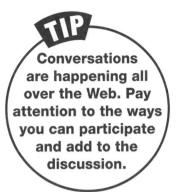

TIP

Conversations are happening all over the Web. Pay attention to the ways you can participate and add to the discussion.

Collaborating

Why do you need to learn about online collaboration?

Although the idea might seem intimidating at first, the potential to collaborate online should be liberating. Using online tools can remove barriers such as different schedules and geographical distance. Also, a number of services can make working on projects easier. And of course, working on research, policy issues, or any special-interest project without these online tools can restrict who you are able to work with. Online collaborative tools enable you to improve how you work with people, whether they work within your organization or are halfway around the world.

What is the benefit of using social media to collaborate online?

Any tool, whether digital or analog, has advantages and disadvantages. Using online collaborative tools helps to overcome some the challenges associated with working with tools that were not designed to do what we need them to do. For example, document-processing software was not designed to provide an easy way to collaborate, and e-mail was not meant for project management. Online, you can use tools designed to enable multiple authors to work on the same presentation at the same time, edit a project in real time, and have meetings without the need to be in the same room.

How can you schedule time to work with other people?

Arranging a time to meet is a regular challenge when working in a group. Fortunately, a few web services provide a way to easily schedule appointments and meeting times online. The following are just two of the options that make it easier to collaborate online:

* Doodle (http://doodle.com)—With this online time-scheduling tool, you can enter a number of potential meeting times and send them to other collaborators.

* Tungle (http://www.tungle.me)—This sophisticated scheduling tool lets you enter your agenda so that others can schedule appointments with you. Using Tungle, a colleague, student, or long-distance collaborator can easily set up a time to meet.

How can you arrange a meeting if people are in different places?

As you've discovered, several online tools are available to help you easily set up meetings. Once the meeting is set up, you can use a free application such as Skype (http://skype.com) to conduct video calls with a person in a different location or to host a voice chat among multiple people. Skype is an easy and free way to work with other nurses, whether they live across town or across the continent. Video and voice chat aren't just great for meetings, they're also fantastic for catching up with old colleagues. And, since Skype is free, it can save you money!

Insights & Inspiration

Rafael Pineda-Perdomo

@rapinedape

http://ideasenfermeria.org

I understand that many nurses are skeptical that technology and social media can benefit nursing. My interest in the area began to grow, however, as I began to see how people from diverse sectors, lifestyles, and professions used these tools in an incredible way. I watched videos about leadership on Harvard Business School's YouTube channel and inspirational talks on TED (http://www.ted.com/), and I found value in blogs created by nurses.

In 2009, I started downloading podcasts from RNL (Reflections on Nursing Leadership magazine, www.reflectionsonnursingleadership.org). In an article published there, I found a website created by Rob Fraser, and I decided to contact him via video chat, using Skype. After that, we communicated through e-mails. I soon found sites such as Twitter, LinkedIn, and Mendeley, where I could connect with nurses around the world and join conversations, share knowledge, and learn what nurses with interests similar to mine were doing around the world. I think that social media can give nurses a greater voice.

I had in mind to do something of my own in the social media space someday, but I couldn't think of a good idea. Then, after reflecting awhile, I talked with Rob about starting a Spanish version of his website, Nursing Ideas (http://nursingideas.ca). I used my technology skills to launch Ideas de Enfermeria, providing a platform for nurses and researchers in health care in Spanish-speaking countries to share their ideas.

Lesson: Many might think that starting a website is difficult and requires advanced knowledge and experience. At the beginning, it did seem rather complex. But then it became more intuitive. Finding a good template and generating good content are usually the keys. Now, 8 months in, Ideas de Enfermeria has been well-received. Many nurses from various regions have been encouraged to participate with comments and discussions. To put it in figures, the site has received about 1,500 visits.

What tools are available for collaborating with other people?

The two main categories of tools for digital collaboration are as follows:

* Wikis—A wiki is a website that enables collaborators to easily add and edit web pages. The most commonly used wiki is Wikipedia (http://wikipedia.org), which allows anyone to add and edit pages on topics of all kinds. Using services such as PBworks (http://pbworks.com), you can create wikis free of charge. This offers a great way to work on group projects online, rather than coordinating activity by e-mail and then trying to piece together all the separate work.

* Web-based document services—Using these services, users can create and edit documents, spreadsheets, and presentations online. The most popular example of this type of service is Google Docs (http://docs.google.com). With Google Docs, multiple individuals can work on the same document, rather than everyone working on separate sections and then combining them at the end.

When is it better to use a wiki versus a shared online document?

Using online collaborative tools involves a bit of a learning curve, as does deciding when to use them. There is no set of rules or decision tree to follow. Instead, you simply need to focus on what you are trying to accomplish. Shared documents are best for producing a document, presentation, or spreadsheet from a collaborative effort. Wikis are meant for larger projects and for organizing activities.

What type of projects can these tools be used for?

Wikis and collaborative documents have myriad functions and capabilities and are not limited to certain types of use. The best way to use them is to learn what they are capable of doing and try them out for different projects. Table 9.1 contains a few ideas about potential uses for wikis and collaborative documents.

Ideal tasks for wikis and collaborative documents

Wiki	Collaborative Document
Project management	Writing a proposal
Organizing unit policies	Creating a conference presentation
Developing an educational course	Developing a unit newsletter
Reviewing practice guidelines	Keeping a group or project budget up to date
Creating unit learning resources	Creating forms and surveys
Collaborating on a research project	Making an agenda for a meeting

Frequently Asked Questions

 How can you make it easier to use social-networking tools?

The key to using social-networking tools effectively is to develop a system. Practice the system, and then improve it. Social media and digital social-networking tools are very new. Simply beginning to use them is a good start, but setting specific goals and purposes enables you to experiment with how you can best use these new tools. The mark of a good tool is its ability to effectively and efficiently complete a task, which is why you need to test these tools yourself to see if they work well for you.

 What is the key to getting a lot of followers or friends?

Although social-networking tools can easily count the number of connections you have, this number is not important. What really matters is your relationship with those individuals and the value you get from using these tools. Instead of focusing on having a large number of connections, concentrate on having strong relationships with the people in your social networks, and make sure the people you are connected with are adding value to your experience.

Is there an easy way to start using collaborative tools?

The best way to learn to use collaborative tools is to experiment with them. Although this may cause you a few headaches, remember that the traditional way of doing things also causes headaches. The only difference is that you forget the problems of a pen until you compare it to a pencil. Remind yourself that the way you used to do things also had its challenges, and that learning new ways to do things can help solve other problems. Start by using tools that solve problems. For example, if you want to connect with a friend abroad but calling another country is too expensive, try using Skype. If you need to schedule a meeting, try using Doodle. The order is not important; what matters is remembering what tools are available and trying them when they appear to solve a problem. If they are successful, you can add them to the list of your digital toolset.

How can you encourage others to try new collaborative tools?

Everyone wants to work more effectively and efficiently, and many people are willing to invest time, if they think it will save them time in the future. Try explaining the benefits, or how you think a tool might be useful to them. When people understand what a web service or social media tool is useful for, they will be more interested in using it. If you cannot convince them, try to understand why they are reluctant. They may not fully understand the tool, or perhaps they feel they cannot learn it on their own. If you really want to use digital collaboration tools, it's best to start with willing and excited partners. Signing others up who are resistant to using a tool will likely create additional challenges that might cause your project to fail, so be sure your collaborators are truly on your side.

Where is this technology heading? What do you need to prepare for?

Similar to cell phones, e-mail, and the first social networks, collaborative tools will, at some point, become tools that most everyone will use. Some may resist and avoid them, but as more people use these tools, it will become everyone's responsibility to learn how to use them in order to build relationships and work effectively with others. As nurses, we need to remember that although we are skilled care providers, we are also knowledge workers. The nursing profession must learn to leverage every tool possible, including social media tools, to develop knowledge more efficiently and share that knowledge with others.

Exercises

1. Talking about networking and collaborating is useful, but the best way to learn how to use these new networking and collaborating tools is to put what you have learned into practice. First, do an assessment to see whether there are ways to improve how you manage your contacts and opportunities for you to benefit from using online tools. Start by asking yourself these questions:

   * Do you have a place to enter and store a person's contact information after you get his or her business card or receive an e-mail from him or her?

   * Have you ever lost track of a person's contact information?

   * Have you ever tried to call or write someone but found that you didn't have up-to-date information for that person?

   * Have you ever used a social-networking tool to find someone you wanted to get in touch with?

* Do you have a plan to regularly get in touch with your friends, family, and colleagues to avoid losing touch with them?

2. If you think you can improve the way you manage your contacts, make a list of what you want to improve, and then consider whether an online tool might help you achieve that goal. Then try using it.

3. To assess your ability to collaborate with others online, first ask yourself these questions:

   * How do you currently schedule times to work with others or to meet with large groups? Is it effective?

   * Does trying to coordinate schedules lead to a large number of e-mails and a struggle to decide on a time to meet?

   * Have you ever found it difficult to work with someone because you couldn't find times to meet in person and were forced to communicate only by e-mail?

   * Do know people you wish you could work with but can't, because they live too far away?

   * Have you ever been frustrated because you couldn't work on a document because someone had not sent you the latest version or completed his or her part?

   * Have you ever struggled to keep up with a project or group because there were too many e-mails to read, and you weren't sure what was happening?

4. If you can identify weaknesses in the way you currently collaborate with others, try to find a digital tool that might help you address the problem. Learn what tools make collaboration easier and experiment with them. Then plan to use a new tool the next time the opportunity comes up.

10

*

Where to From Here?

Do you:

Understand the different levels of online interaction?

Know what technology experts are highlighting as the important parts of social media?

Recognize how you can use social media for career development, research, and sharing content?

Realize there are different approaches to using social media?

As you've learned, social media is more than just signing up for a social network. Social media changes how we communicate to create exciting new possibilities. But what do those possibilities look like? If social media isn't about the social network, then what is it about? Unfortunately, social media is still relatively new, so there are no clear, simple answers to these questions. Even so, there are tons of great ideas on how to use and get value out of social media.

"A rock pile ceases to be a rock pile the moment a single man contemplates it, bearing within him the image of a cathedral."

–Antoine de Saint-Exupéry

Using Social Media

What do the experts have to say?

There are many books about social media. Many of the ideas in these books have inspired educators, academics, and clinicians to adopt these tools for their own use. Even if these books are written by and for people outside your field, it's important to see others' perspectives on how social media is useful, decide whether this perspective aligns with yours, and determine whether you can learn any lessons from this perspective in terms of how you can use social media.

Following are a few books to consider:

* *Tribes: We Need You to Lead Us* (2008), by Seth Godin—In his book, marketer Seth Godin writes about how the ways we gather audiences are changing. He explores how the Internet enables people with shared values, ideas, and beliefs to assemble. Anyone who has a cause worth pursuing can attract others to that cause. In the past, companies could simply buy more ads to get to the top. In the age of social media, you don't need as much in the way of mass media, but you need more in the way of critical media. When you use critical media, the true believers will take on your cause or find what you are doing is useful. According to Godin, we all can be tribe leaders—sharing important information and ideas that matter to a targeted audience.

* *Trust Agents: Using the Web to Build Influence, Improve Reputation, and Earn Trust* (2009), by Chris Brogan and Julien

Smith—This book explains the power of social media, discussing how anyone can participate online. As business developers and marketers, the authors focus on how businesses can produce great content, engage with people, and have conversations online. The key lesson, though, is that developing your brand takes trust. If people feel that you are engaging with them on the Web to take advantage of them, that you do not respect them, or that you are being selfish, they will peg you as an outsider. Take time to listen, to fit in, and to see how you can add value; don't just sell something or try to be the leader of the pack. Earn trust, the ultimate currency, by getting to know and contributing to your community.

* *Crush It! Why Now Is the Time to Cash in on Your Passion* (2009), by Gary Vaynerchuk—Wine connoisseur Gary Vaynerchuk is one of the most influential voices in social media. His story is compelling not because he knows social media (although he does), but because he used social media to further his passion. When Vaynerchuk took over his family's wine store in New Jersey, he increased sales from $6 million per year to $60 million by engaging people online. The thesis of his book is that through social media, individuals can develop online resources on any subject at an extremely low cost, which can drive sales. His formula: Spend 10% of your time making your product, and 90% engaging your audience.

* *The New Community Rules: Marketing on the Social Web* (2009), by Tamara Weinberg—The main message of this hands-on guide for marketers is that the marketing world has changed. The tools people use are different. Weinberg believes that anyone who understands the tools and the possibilities can begin to engage with them; to that end, she explains the various tools in a very simple way. Although making the leap to using these tools may involve a bit of a shift, anyone can go from zero to hero if he or she dedicates time to learning how the new Web works.

* *The Networked Nonprofit* (2010), by Beth Kanter and Allison H. Fine—This book, aimed at helping nonprofits understand

how they can use social media, focuses on three major themes: social culture, transparency, and simplicity. To use social media within an organization, you must have a culture that supports it, and you must be transparent about your intentions, goals, and aspirations. This approach helps people relate to and identify with your organization. It also enables you to listen when people are upset. An important message of this book is to avoid trying to do too much. Focus on what you do, and ask for help with the rest. Clearly, you can accomplish a lot with social media—and not just selling more widgets. Bringing awareness to social causes and nonprofits is a fantastic example of the good that social media can do!

Just because most of these books focus on using social media for marketing purposes doesn't mean the lessons they contain don't apply to nurses!

What are some practical ways nurses can use social media?

Following are some of the ways nurses can use social media:

* For career development

* For research

* To share content and collaborate

These are just some of the ways nurses can use social media. Each person brings a different perspective that can create new uses for social media! Hopefully, what you read here will inspire you to try these tools in new ways.

Career Development

How can nurses use social media for career development?

In terms of career development, nurses can use social media in the following ways:

To engage the public

To market themselves

To build and manage relationships

To make and measure their impact

How can nurses use social media to engage the public?

One of my heroes is journalist Suzanne Gordon (2010), who preaches that "nurses are not articulating their work and putting their brain—as opposed to their hearts—in the forefront of their conversation" (para. 1). Gordon believes nurses should talk about their lifesaving knowledge and skills. Social media is a great platform for nurses to share their expertise with the public and to shed insight into what nurses do and the value they add to the health care system.

How can nurses use social media to market themselves?

Nursing education doesn't typically include coursework on marketing yourself, but it should. The fact is, individuals, whatever their line of work, need to be able to clearly communicate what their skills are, what makes them unique, and how they can contribute to society—essentially, to brand themselves much the same way companies do (Peters, 1997). Fortunately, nursing leaders such as Waddell, Donner, and Wheeler (2009) have begun encouraging nurses to create a vision for their careers and to take steps to achieve it. Along with performing an environmental scan and a self-assessment and engaging in strategic planning, they highly encourage nurses to find ways to market themselves.

Social media offers nurses a perfect way to do this. Amy Sellers' web page, http://amysellers.me, is a great example of a professional online portfolio. This simple but effective page was created by nurse Amy Sellers to share a bit of personal and professional information. It, along with her blog, Nursing Influence (http://nursinginfluence.com) is a great marketing tool.

How can nurses use social media to build and manage relationships?

Knowing the CEO of your hospital is one thing; being able to approach that person is something else entirely. One of the best things about social media is that anyone who joins a social network and publicly shares information is literally asking to be approached about those topics. That really opens the door for communicating, collaborating, and sharing resources—and you just never know how these could positively affect your career down the road. In my case, a conversation I had on Twitter had numerous unplanned effects on my career, including being featured in magazines and presenting at conferences, not to mention writing the book you are reading right now!

TIP

You can use LinkedIn to search for individuals or groups related to your nursing specialty or area of interest.

How can nurses use social media to make and measure their impact?

Many nurses have valuable experiences and ideas to share. Publishing peer-reviewed papers and books, however, may not necessarily be the best way to make an impact. Why not try creating a blog or video channel? Using the World Wide Web—especially with the advent of Web 2.0—to share valuable information with other nurses gives them an opportunity to credit you for your work and link back to your original content. To measure your impact, simply measure the number of views, links, and comments on your content.

Researching

How can nurses use social media for research?

In terms of research, nurses can use social media for the following:

Finding content

Organizing content

Obtaining feedback

How can nurses use social media to find content?

Many nurses are researching very important and relevant issues. Traditional literature is no longer the only source for information, however. Being able to search for and find content online greatly expedites this research. From presentations or brochures to clinical tips and literature searches, nurses are starting to post more information online to make it available for others. Using social media sites such as SlideShare (http://slideshare.net), where users can post and download PowerPoint presentations, and YouTube (http://youtube.com) helps nurses find materials on their topic of interest.

TIP

Researchers call unpublished work *grey literature*, meaning it is not from traditional channels.

How can nurses use social media to organize content?

Using social media is a great way to keep up with changing trends in health care and to share that information with others. Just as sticky notes and binders help you keep information organized in the real world, many social media tools can help you organize your online content. Tags, social bookmarks, and filters are all great examples of organization features that social media applications offer. Other examples include tools that enable you to annotate PDF files and to create research collections, which is helpful for keeping all your articles in one place.

How can nurses use social media to obtain feedback?

Publishing articles in research journals can take months or even years—and the time it takes for others to register their feedback through traditional channels can be even longer. In contrast, using a blog as a research journal, sharing literature searches online, or entering status updates on social networks can allow others to give instant feedback. I've experienced this firsthand on many occasions. For example, one time I was working on a research project when a status update led me to Kevin Clauson (http://twitter.com/kevinclauson), who sent me a search he had done a few weeks earlier. On another occasion, while working on a policy update for a hospital, I used Twitter to ask how nurses checked nasogastric tubes at their hospitals; 25 nurses responded within minutes. Getting feedback can be very helpful for developing ideas and ensuring that nothing is left out.

Sharing Content and Collaborating

TIP

Increasing the speed of research can help nurses learn from each other how to improve patient care.

How can nurses use social media to share content?

If your résumé, or your research on the latest techniques in your area of interest, is safely hidden in your desk drawer, how is anyone (except you, of course) ever going to find it? Using social media is a great way to help extend the life of your work and expertise. Whether it's a nursing portfolio or a presentation that you regularly deliver, posting content online helps you spread ideas faster, so that others can find what they are looking for—and the expert who created it.

What are the benefits of using social media to share content?

Social media can breathe new life into material that otherwise sits unused. Take Home Depot as an example. Home Depot has begun posting videos of tutorials the company gives in-store on YouTube (http://www.youtube.com/user/homedepot). This online content doesn't replace what the company is doing in stores; it merely extends the life of that content. Both avenues help Home Depot accomplish its goal of helping customers learn how to use the products they sell. Ask yourself: What is your hospital's goal? What is your goal? Are you giving patients information in person that they could also review online, or information that patients elsewhere might find beneficial?

How can nurses use social media to collaborate?

Social media is more than just connecting online and creating new opportunities. All sorts of social media tools can make collaboration easier and cheaper. For example, nurses can use Skype (http://www.skype.com) to call or video chat with other nurses around the world—for free. And, nurses in different rooms or on different continents can use document-editing tools such as Google Docs (http://docs.google.com) to work on shared documents.

Numerous Opportunities

Why are there so many different perspectives on how to use social media?

Every social media network, service, and tool has a different function. More importantly, it's used by different people. Take the photo-sharing site Flickr (http://flickr.com) as an example. Two different people—even two different nurses—might post their photos on Flickr for very different reasons. One might post photos from a conference she attended to share them with colleagues. This serves to build and strengthen relationships and to promote her image by demonstrating professional involvement. The other nurse might post photos of the same conference and share them with conference organizers in attempt to market herself for future events.

The fact is, everyone comes to social networking sites with a different purpose in mind. We look at social media the way we look at a tree. Even if we are all examining the same tree, our height, our vision, and our position relative to the tree shape our perspective of that tree. Similarly, your experience, knowledge, and goals shape how you see social media and what you might choose to do with it.

"Everyone sees a different tree."

–Mr. Horton, my 11th-grade English teacher

Is there something people do agree on?

Although there's no real consensus on why individuals do what they do online, there is emerging evidence of what people do online. Singh, Lehnert, and Bostick (2010) surveyed 3,800 social media users to find out why they were using social media. The study found that the top business-related social media activities were as follows:

* Building networks

* Consuming content (reading articles, watching videos or presentations, etc.)

* Demonstrating personal and professional expertise

In addition, the study determined that the top personal social media activities were as follows:

* Connecting with family and friends

* Consuming content (reading articles, looking at pictures, watching videos, etc.)

* Finding like-minded people (hobbies, interests, political views, etc.)

* Sharing links with others

* Making new friends

Another great survey (Li, Bernoff, Fiorentino, & Glass, 2007) shows how adults and teens are slowly integrating different functions of social media into their lives (see Figure 10.1).

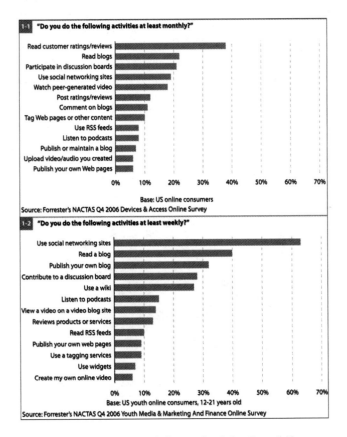

Figure 10.1: Many people use the Internet, but their online activities vary.

As you can see, there are many different ways to engage in social media. In developing your purpose for using social media, ask yourself: Where should I start? How can I be intentional?

Making Progress

How do users get started?

In my experience, users generally start with social media by using the first service to which they are introduced. For example, a person might learn to post video blogs but have no idea how to find nursing podcasts. For nurses who are looking to get involved, I suggest starting either by thinking about what you want to do or, if you are a bit intimidated by the technology, about how you can slowly immerse yourself.

What are the phases of social media use?

Figure 10.2 shows the various phases of social media use, as conceptualized by Li, Bernoff, Fiorentino, and Glass (2007).

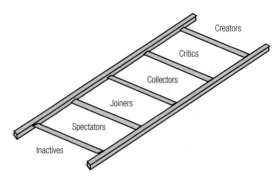

Figure 10.2: The Consumer Activity Ladder (Li et al., 2007).

The phases are as follows:

* Inactives—People in this first stage account for 52% of the adult online population (Li et al., 2007). They tend to think their opinion is not worth sharing and do not consider themselves leaders.

* Spectators—Spectators make up 33% of the population of adults who are online (Li et al., 2007). People in this group consume content developed by peers.

* Joiners—Joiners are the adult crowd that has begun participating online by joining social networks. These users account for 19% of active online adults (Li et al., 2007).

* Collectors—Collectors include people who use social bookmarking and tagging. These activities benefit users by making information more accessible. According to Li et al. (2007), 15% of online adults fit into this category.

* Critics—While critics may seem like a derogatory term, it simply refers to people who listen, observe, and then share their opinions. Just as a theater critic watches a production and offers praise or criticism, these digital critics take in blogs, videos, and other content and leave comments, ratings, and reviews. This group encompasses about 19% of online adults (Li et al., 2007).

* Creators—Found at the top of the ladder, creators comprise the smallest group—only 13% of adults online (Li et al., 2007). Participants in this group upload content to a blog, website, or video channel on a monthly basis.

This model provides a simple way to think about participation. The downside of this model is that because of its ladder structure, it perhaps places too much emphasis on the top, suggesting that creators are the most important group. Li and colleagues do mention that some online participants might fit into multiple groups. Although becoming active is important, it's more important to purposefully and meaningfully progress when learning to use social media tools.

For nurses—or anyone, for that matter—moving from the inactive group to the creator group is a big leap. More importantly, it is intimidating.

How can nurses think about engaging?

Being a spectator is one way to learn, but I would like to propose another approach to engaging in social media. In my view, you can use social media for nine basic activities (see Figure 10.3). Hopefully, they are all activities you are already doing offline.

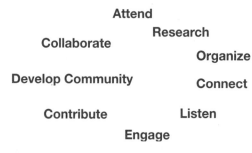

Attend

Research

Collaborate

Organize

Develop Community

Connect

Contribute

Listen

Engage

Figure 10.3: You can use social media for nine basic activities.

These are the basic components of becoming a social media power user. This is not to imply, however, that any one of these activities or phases is the best. Some activities will come easier than others and, at times, you may switch among them. For example, sometimes you may spend more time contributing than listening, and other times the opposite will be true.

What happens in the Attend phase?

This activity involves simply setting up a profile on LinkedIn or Facebook. Even if you do nothing more than enter your basic information, others can find you and link to your profile. Although you may also have your own web page on your hospital's or university's website, a profile you can control is better, because you have the power to update it if you develop a new interest or area of expertise.

What happens in the Research phase?

To search through the ever-growing amount of information on the Web, you must have the ability to do research. This capacity includes knowing the different search tools and being able to set up search alerts. When you participate in social media, you must be able to locate all sorts of information, ranging from people with similar clinical interests to experts who are sharing certain types of information to specific content that you need.

What happens in the Organize phase?

Humans can memorize only so much information. After perusing any more than a few web pages, you are bound to forget what you read a few pages earlier—especially in a community that continually posts new conversations, develops new material, and shares new resources. Social bookmarking, tagging, organizing, setting up subscriptions, and creating mail filters help you to deal with the increase in information.

What happens in the Connect phase?

If you think of the first three stages as building the foundation, you can think of connecting as hooking up the power. Connecting—following, adding, linking, or whatever term social media sites use—is what powers social media. Sharing information with anyone, whether family, friends, colleagues, coworkers, or others interested in similar topics, unleashes the power of the Internet.

What happens in the Listen phase?

When joining any group, it's considered courteous to listen before you speak. When you find individuals and communities that are creating and discussing content that interests you, don't jump in with your opinions right away. Take some time to observe the activity on the site first.

What happens in the Engage phase?

After you learn the norms of any site or group, the next step is to respectfully begin to participate. Contributing to conversations and sharing additional ideas and experiences through comments or on Twitter are easy ways to begin building relationships, knowledge, and trust online.

What happens in the Contribute phase?

In this phase, you take time to develop and contribute content beyond commenting and social bookmarking. Depending on the content and your preferences for communicating, these contributions might be text, pictures, videos, or audio. This phase is more about quality and consistency than frequency.

What happens in the Develop Community phase?

Too often, organizers and even individuals want to be leaders—the first to create a new social network for nurses. Social media is about community, however. It's not about who founded a particular site. Sometimes, there will be legitimate reasons to create a new place to converse and share online. But, you should always check to see if this is already being done somewhere. If it is, find ways to strengthen those efforts. Instead of focusing on how to start a community, think about how to build or contribute to existing ones.

What happens in the Collaborate phase?

Once you start using social media tools to interact with others online, and teaching your colleagues about social media tools offline, find ways to use them. Maybe that means using document-editing tools that make writing and editing easier, or using Skype to video conference with a nurse in another state or country who shares your interest. These tools are meant to be used to develop and create. As the saying goes, "Two heads are better than one."

Do you have to use them all at once?

One of the big misconceptions about social networking is that it will consume all your time. It does not have to. To prevent this, remember two important things:

* Small investments over time add up to big results—It's better to slowly grow and develop than to dedicate large amounts of time and then burn yourself out.

* You can create a plan for how you want to use social media— For example, you might dedicate 30 minutes every other day to a social networking site to connect with friends and colleagues. Or, once a month, you might write about a good research article or share a practice insight on your blog.

If your goal is to develop a credible professional online presence over the course of your career, quality beats quantity every time.

Frequently Asked Questions

 Is it necessary to have your own website?

By the end of this book, you will have at least a few websites—specifically, the profiles and pages you set up on various social-networking sites. But, you don't have to buy or host your own domain. And don't worry, you won't need to become a Web developer or learn code!

 If you do not have a business, do you need to use social media?

Do you have any passions that you want to share with others? Do you want to connect with others who share your interests? Social media can be a great way to do just that. Social media can also help you stay up to date with new research and information on topics that interest you. And, of course, having a strong network and personal brand can help you find new opportunities as your career takes new and unexpected turns.

What is the benefit of joining LinkedIn?

LinkedIn is a professional networking site. On it, you can share your profile (similar to a résumé), manage relationships with colleagues, follow companies, and join groups. Joining it can be very beneficial for anyone who wants to expand professionally.

If you're feeling overwhelmed, how should you get started?

First, take a deep breath. You wouldn't try to learn how to figure skate by watching the Winter Olympics. Instead, you'd begin by breaking things down into small steps—crawl before you walk, walk before you run. The same is true with learning to use social media. If you have friends or colleagues who use social media, why not ask them to give you a bit of help? Start with one site and slowly learn the features before moving on to the next. Don't expect perfection; just continue to learn and improve what you are doing.

TIP

If you're not sure whether you want to join a site, read its description online to understand the benefits of joining.

Does social media replace offline relationships?

Social media does not replace offline relationships. Think of it this way: You don't typically phone someone when he or she is in the same room, but a telephone does give you the ability to talk to people who are far away. The fact is, nurses need to develop their careers both offline and online. Using online services is beneficial because you can connect more regularly with passionate and engaged nurses whom you might normally see only once a year at a conference. Use these tools to keep in contact, but continue to build relationships offline too.

If you have a good job that you plan to keep for a long time, why do you need social media?

In today's economy, and as the health care industry continues to experience tremendous changes, cutbacks can occur. That means every nurse needs a backup plan. Besides, social media offers a lot in the way of possibilities. If you're a nurse with years on the job, you have a lot of experience that could benefit new graduates. Why not use social media to share your expertise before you leave the workplace? Or, maybe your hospital needs to update policies or find new ways to improve clinical care. In that case, keeping in touch with other professionals in different organizations is a great way to discover what innovations they are pursuing to improve client care.

Exercises

1. Start with yourself. Pull out the latest copy of your résumé; then write down what you think others might say about you professionally. This is your brand. If you like it, great! If not, you can change it.

2. To change your brand, begin by thinking about what you want your brand to be. Ask yourself these questions:

   * What is your expertise?

   * What are you passionate about?

   * In five sentences or less, what do you want other people to know about you?

   * What knowledge could you share that would benefit others?

   * What are your career goals? What do you need to do, and who do you need to work with, to achieve them?

3. Write down which benefits of using social media appeal to you. As you continue learning about social media, keep them in mind. When you encounter new social media tools, consider whether they offer these benefits. If not, could you use

them to accomplish other goals that would build your brand
and create value for others?

4. Go online and, taking into account both your expertise and
how you want to use social media, use Google.com to search
for websites, blogs, and videos that relate to your area of expertise and your interests. Do you find any content—blogs,
videos, presentations, etc.—from nurses? Surveying the landscape can identify gaps for you to fill or identify role models
for you to follow.

A

References

Frontmatter

Martin, G.Z. (2010). 30 Days to Social Media Success. Pompton: Career Press, 2010.

Wikipedia. "Social Media," 2010. http://en.wikipedia.org/w/index. php?title=Social_media&oldid=266390217.

Chapter 1

Barrientos, F., & Foughty, E. (2009). Web 2.0 in government. *Interactions, 16*(5), 29–35.

Bylund, A. (2006, 5 July). To google or not to google. The Motley Fool. Retrieved 1 January 2011 from http://www.fool.com/investing/ dividends-income/2006/07/05/to-google-or-not-to-google.aspx

Fox, S. (2007, 8 October). E-patients with a disability or chronic disease. Pew Internet & American Life Project. Retrieved 1 January 2011 from http://www.pewinternet.org/Reports/2007/Epatients-With-a-Disability-or-Chronic-Disease.aspx

Fox, S. (2008, 6 March). Recruit doctors. Let e-patients lead. Go mobile. Pew Internet & American Life Project. Retrieved 1 January 2011 from http://e-patients.net/archives/2008/03/recruit-doctors-let-e-patients-lead-go-mobile.html

Governor, J., Nickull, D., & Hinchcliffe, D. (2009). Web 2.0 architectures. Cambridge, MA: O'Reilly Media.

Horrigan, J. B., & Rainie, L. (2002, 29 December). Counting on the Internet: Most find the information they seek, expect. Pew Internet & American Life Project. Retrieved 1 January 2011 from http://www.pewinternet.org/Reports/2002/Counting-on-the-Internet-Most-find-the-information-they-seek-expect.aspx

Kreps, G., Beckjord, E. Atkinson, N. L., Saperstein, S. L., & Pleis, J. (2009). Using the Internet for health-related activities: Finding a national probability sample. Journal of Medical Internet Research, 11(1), e4. DOI:10.2196/jmir.1035

O'Reilly, T. (2005, 30 September). What is Web 2.0: Design patterns and business models for the next generation of software. O'Reilly Media. Retrieved 1 January 2011 from http://oreilly.com/web2/archive/what-is-web-20.html

Shirky, C. (2009). How social media can make history. Video of presentation at TED Conference. Retrieved 1 January 2011 from http://www.ted.com/talks/clay_shirky_how_cellphones_twitter_facebook_can_make_history.html

Smith, A. (2010, 11 August). Home broadband 2010. Pew Internet & American Life Project. Retrieved 1 January 2011 from http://www.pewinternet.org/Reports/2010/Home-Broadband-2010.aspx

Chapter 3

American Medical Association. (2010, 10 November). AMA policy: Professionalism in the use of social media. Retrieved 1 January 2011 from http://www.ama-assn.org/ama/pub/meeting/professionalism-social-media.shtml

Dolan, P. L. (2008, 2 June). Social networking etiquette: Making virtual acquaintances. American Medical News. Retrieved 1 January 2011 from http://www.ama-assn.org/amednews/2008/06/02/bisa0602.htm

Dolan, P. L. (2009, 12 October). Social media behavior could threaten your reputation, job prospects. Journal of the American Medical Association. Retrieved 1 January 2011 from http://www.ama-assn.org/amednews/2009/10/12/bil21012.htm

Givens, L. (2009, 6 August). Libel and social media. Black Web Media. Retrieved 1 January 2011 from http://www.blackweb20.com/2009/08/06/libel-and-social-media/

O'Reilly, K. B. (2010, 6 September). Social media pose ethical unknowns for doctors. American Medical News. Retrieved 1 January 2011 from http://www.ama-assn.org/amednews/2010/09/06/prl20906.htm

Ressler, P. K., & Glazer, G. (2010, 22 October). Legislative: Nursing's engagement in health policy and healthcare through social media. Online Journal of Issues in Nursing, 16(1). Retrieved 1 January 2011 from http://www.nursingworld.org/MainMenuCategories/ANAMarketplace/ANAPeriodicals/OJIN/TableofContents/Vol-16-2011/No1-Jan-2011/Health-Policy-and-Healthcare-Through-Social-Media.aspx

Chapter 4

Baker, M., & Lilly, J. (2010, 22 February). Web browser choice matters. OpenToChoice. Retrieved 1 January 2011 from http://opentochoice.org/2010/02/web-browser-choice-matters/

Gube, J. (2009, 14 October). Performance comparison of major web browsers. Six Revisions. Retrieved 1 January 2011 from http://sixrevisions.com/infographics/performance-comparison-of-major-web-browsers/

Krebs, B. (2007, 4 January). Internet Explorer unsafe for 284 days in 2006. The Washington Post. Retrieved 1 January 2011 from http://blog.washingtonpost.com/securityfix/2007/01/internet_explorer_unsafe_for_2.html

Rainie, L., Estabrook, L., & Witt, E. (2007, 30 December). Information searches that solve problems. Pew Internet & American Life Project. Retrieved 1 January 2011 from http://www.pewinternet.org/Reports/2007/Information-Searches-That-Solve-Problems.aspx

Smith, A. (2010a, 7 July). Mobile access 2010. Pew Internet & American Life Project. Retrieved 1 January 2011 from http://www.pewinternet.org/Reports/2010/Mobile-Access-2010.aspx

Smith, A. (2010b, 11 August). Home broadband 2010. Pew Internet & American Life Project. Retrieved 1 January 2011 from http://www.pewinternet.org/Reports/2010/Home-Broadband-2010.aspx

StatsCounter. (2010, November). Global stats: November 2009 to November 2010. Retrieved 1 January 2011 from http://gs.statcounter.com/#browser-ww-monthly-200911-201011

Chapter 5

Covey, S. (2004). The 7 habits of highly effective people. New Jersey: Free Press.

Mann, M. (2007). Original Inbox Zero video. Retrieved 20 January 2009 from http://inboxzero.com/video

Pausch, R. (2007). Time management. Retrieved 1 January 2011 from http://www.youtube.com/watch?v=oTugjssqOT0

Shirky, C. (2008). It's not information overload. It's filter failure. Web 2.0 Expo. Retrieved 1 January 2011 from http://blip.tv/file/1277460

Xplane. (2009). Did you know? Version 4.0. Retrieved 1 January 2011 from http://www.youtube.com/watch?v=6ILQrUrEWe8&feature=related

Chapter 6

Alvarez del Blanco, R. (2010). Personal brands: Manage your life with talent and turn it into a unique experience. Hampshire, England: Palgrave Macmillan.

Chapter 7

Baumann, P. (2009, 18 January). 140 health care uses for Twitter. Phil Baumann. Retrieved 1 January 2011 from http://philbaumann. com/2009/01/18/free-ebook-140-health-care-uses-for-twitter/

Mann, K., Gordon, J., & MacLeod, A. (2009). Reflection and reflective practice in health professions education: A systematic review. Advances in Health Sciences Education: Theory and Practice, 14(4), 595–621.

Oermann, M. H., & Hays, J. C. (2002). Writing for publication in nursing (2nd ed.). New York: Springer.

Rizo, C., Deshpande, A., Ing, A., & Seeman, N. (2010, 12 August). A rapid, web-based method for obtaining patient views on effects and side-effects of antidepressants. Journal of Affective Disorders. DOI: 10.1016.j.jad.2010.07.027

Sullivan-Marx, E., McGivern, D., Fairman, J., & Greensberg, A. (2010). The evolution and future of advanced practice. New York: Springer.

Chapter 8

Aaker, J., & Smith, A. (2010). The dragonfly effect: Quick, effective, and powerful ways to use social media to drive social change. San Francisco: Jossey-Bass.

Chapter 9

Lavrusik, V. (2010, 6 December). Commenting guidelines for the Mashable community. Mashable. Retrieved 1 January 2011 from http:// mashable.com/2010/12/06/commenting-guidelines-for-the-mashable-community/

Chapter 10

Gordon, S. (2010, 15 October). Nursing and the perils of success. Suzanne Gordon. Retrieved 1 January 2011 from http://www. suzannegordon.com/?p=460

Li, C., Bernoff, J., Fiorentino, R., & Glass, S. (2007). Social technographics: Mapping participation in activities forms the foundation of a social strategy. Cambridge, MA: Forrester Research.

Peters, T. (1997). The brand called you. Fast Company. Retrieved 1 January 2011 from http://www.fastcompany.com/magazine/10/brandyou. html

Singh, N., Lehnert, K., & Bostick, K. (2010). Global social media usage and the language factor. Waltham, MA: Lionbridge.

Waddell, J., Donner, G., & Wheeler, M. (2009). Building your nursing career: A guide for students. Toronto, Canada: Mosby Elsevier.

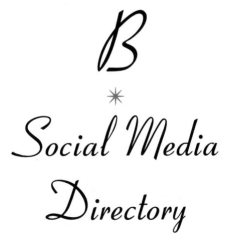

B

Social Media Directory

Analytics, URL Shortening, and Tracking Services

* Snipurl (http://snipurl.com)—Use this free site to shorten long and unmemorable URLs. It offers customizable endings and keeps statistics on how many people click your link.

* Su.pr (http://su.pr)—This free URL-shortening site places linked pages into a website promotion service to help increase traffic. It easily integrates with Twitter to post links and provides feedback on the most effective time to post links based on clicks and responses.

* Bit.ly (http://bit.ly)—This free service enables users to shorten, share, and track links. Integration with Twitter and Facebook is possible.

* Google Analytics (http://google.com/analytics)—Use this free service to collect visitor information for websites, such as the traffic source (referral, search, etc.) and time on the site.

* HootSuite (http://hootsuite.com)—This site, which is free but offers additional services for a fee, enables you to manage and track links you share via your Twitter account and to automatically tweet content from an RSS feed (i.e., your blog).

Bookmarking, Note-Taking, and Organizing

* Delicious (http://delicious.com)—This free site makes bookmarking easy. You simply use the site's browser extension or copy and paste a URL to bookmark a site.

* Diigo (http://www.diigo.com)—Ever wish you could highlight text or make a note on a web page? Now you can, using Diigo's simple and free browser add-on. With Diigo, you can save notes and highlights in your personal (private) or shared (public) library.

* Evernote (http://evernote.com)—This site, which is free but offers additional services for a fee, is like a digital notebook: You can upload text, web clippings, photos, video, and voice notes from your computer or mobile phone. You can tag notes and organize them into folders to make them easier to find.

Blog Services

* WordPress (http://wordpress.com)—WordPress is an open-source content-management system (CMS) that is a powerful blogging tool. It offers a number of plug-ins and themes free of charge, as well as some premium options for very reasonable prices.

* Tumblr (http://www.tumblr.com)—This blogging service is free, but offers additional options for a fee. It focuses on design and simplicity. The service is easy to set up, use, and maintain, but it offers little in the way of options.

* Posterous (http://posterous.com)—This free service makes blogging as easy as sending an e-mail to post@posterous.com. When you send the e-mail, the site adds a post to your blog using the e-mail subject as the title and the message as the blog content. Attachments (images, movies, audio, etc.) are automatically compressed and embedded. You can also use Posterous to post content on Twitter and Facebook.

* Blogger (http://blogger.com)—This free blogging service from Google offers easy integration with Gmail accounts and has very good spam filters.

* TypePad (http://typepad.com)—This fee-based blogging service has a wide variety of themes to choose from. Also, TypePad will handle buying and hosting your blog's domain name (for example, nurseexample.com) for a low price. A free trial is available.

* LiveJournal (http://livejournal.com)—This blogging service, which is free but offers additional options for a fee, focuses on journaling and self-expression. It specializes in blogs for groups that wish to share information privately. It's not highly encrypted but does support sophisticated password options.

Collaboration and File Sharing

* Google Docs (http://docs.google.com)—Use Google Docs to create, edit, and share documents, spreadsheets, and presentations free of charge. Instead of e-mailing different versions of a document, you can use Google Docs for live, simultaneous editing from different computers.

* Docs (http://docs.com)—Docs is Microsoft and Facebook's free competitor to Google Docs. It's great for sharing Word, Excel, and PowerPoint files for research and collaboration.

* Dropbox (http://dropbox.net)—Use this site to automatically back up and sync files. For example, you can use this service to ensure that when you save a file to a folder at work, it's automatically saved to your laptop as well. You can also use the site, which is free but offers additional fee-based options, to share folders with other users or to transfer files that are too large for e-mail.

* SlideShare (http://slideshare.net)—Use this service, which is free but offers additional fee-based options, to upload and share PowerPoint files and to record audio for slides. It's perfect for sharing presentations, thereby building your reputation as an expert.

* Skype (http://skype.com)—Skype uses Voice over IP (VoIP) technology to offer users free calling and video chat anywhere they have access to the Internet. It works well for meetings with people in different locations.

* PBworks (http://pbworks.com)—PBworks offers tiered wiki services for clients, ranging from personal to organizational. It supports collaborative knowledge and resource building in a private or open environment.

Microblogs

* FriendFeed (http://friendfeed.com)—This free site offers aggregation services, pulling in user activity on social media sites, and also a microblogging feature.

* Twitter (http://twitter.com)—Use Twitter to share information with others in short bursts (there's a 140-character limit). For example, you might indicate what you are doing, working on, or reading. It's useful for keeping up with friends and for following content providers (CNN, BBC, American Journal of Nursing, etc.).

News Aggregators and Channels

* Alltop (http://nursing.alltop.com)—This free service aggregates RSS feeds from nursing websites. You can use it to easily browse titles of recent articles to find what interests you. You can also submit your own RSS feed, so others can find your articles.

* Digg (http://digg.com)—You can use Digg, a sort of curated free news source, to share bookmarks and vote on stories. Articles with higher ratings appear first. You can also follow users with similar interests.

* Google Reader (http://google.com/reader)—Google provides this RSS feed aggregator free of charge. You can use it to add RSS feeds, follow friends' recommendations, and easily share articles you find interesting.

* iGoogle (http://google.com/ig)—This free, customizable website can display local weather, news, RSS feeds of interest, daily trivia, and so on. It's like a dashboard of useful information. You can use iGoogle as a home page, rather than visiting individual websites.

* Netvibes (http://netvibes.com)—This free site is a self-proclaimed "Dashboard for Everything." You can use it to create a nursing-related dashboard. Netvibes will then pull in news, pictures, and videos that relate to nursing. Additional customization is possible, as are subscriptions to specific websites.

Picture Sharing and Search

* Compfight (http://compfight.com)—Use this free site to easily search Creative Commons photographs—for example, to find a photograph of pills for a presentation on administering medication.

* Flickr (http://flickr.com)—Flickr is the largest picture-sharing site, enabling users to upload very high-quality photos (500 for free) to share with others. You can also search for and download Creative Commons-licensed pictures to use on your website or in presentations.

* Picasa (http://picasa.google.com)—This free photo-storage and editing service enables you to upload and edit photos, and then share them with friends and family.

* Stock.XCHNG (http://sxc.hu)—Use this free search engine to find Creative Commons-licensed photographs. It's another great resource for finding pictures to illustrate ideas in blog posts or presentations.

Social Sites

* Facebook (http://facebook.com)—Facebook is the largest social network. It enables users to create personal profile pages, group pages, and fan pages (for brands and organizations).

* LinkedIn (http://linkedin.com)—On this professional social-networking site, you can upload your résumé, identify your expertise, and create groups and company profiles.

* Ning (http://ning.com)—Ning lets you create your own social-networking site. It's great for groups that want a private platform or for an organizationally branded network.

Twitter and Social Media Applications

* TweetDeck (http://tweetdeck.com)—This is a free application for your computer or mobile phone (iPhone and BlackBerry) for managing your Twitter account(s).

* OpenBeak (http://www.orangatame.com/products/openbeak/)—This free application for BlackBerry phones enables users to post text, pictures, and videos to Twitter.

* Seesmic (http://seesmic.com)—Use this free desktop client and mobile phone application to manage your Twitter and Facebook account(s). It's ideal for managing different accounts and monitoring multiple Twitter lists.

Video Sharing

* Blip (http://blip.tv)—This site is a video repository. It offers revenue sharing through advertisement. You can use Blip to distribute video to iTunes to reach more people.

* Howcast (http://howcast.com)—This free site specializes in short videos that teach users how to do something, from baking a pie to properly ironing a shirt. Nurses could use this site to demonstrate, for example, head-to-toe assessments or how to set up an IV pump.

* TubeMogul (http://tubemogul.com)—You can use this distribution site to upload a video and then cross-post it to your other accounts (Blip.tv, YouTube, etc.). This can save a lot of time. TubeMogul enables you to place the video in more places, so users can find your content.

* Vimeo (http://vimeo.com)—This site specializes in sharing HD videos. Basic services are free for a limited number of uploaded videos per week. Premium members can upload and stream more HD video.

* YouTube (http://youtube.com)—On YouTube, Google's video channel, video uploads are unlimited and free, although videos cannot exceed 10 minutes. Advertisements are placed on and beside the video. This site boasts the largest user base, meaning users have more opportunity to search for topics related to your video.

Index